Rapid Interpretation of Ventilator Waveforms

Jonathan B. Waugh, Ph.D., RRT, CPFT
Vijay M. Deshpande, M.S., RRT
Robert J. Harwood, M.S.A., RRT

Georgia State University
Cardiopulmonary Care Sciences
Atlanta, Georgia

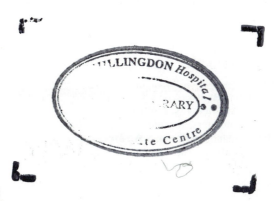
Prentice Hall
Prentice Hall
Upper Saddle River, New Jersey 07458

Publisher: *Susan Katz*
Acquisitions Editor: *Mark Cohen*
Editorial Assistant: *Stephanie Camangian*
Marketing Manager: *Tiffany Price*
Marketing Coordinator: *Cindy Frederick*
Director of Production and Manufacturing: *Bruce Johnson*
Managing Production Editor: *Patrick Walsh*
Production Editor: *Julie Boddorf*
Manufacturing Buyer: *Ilene Sanford*
Printer and Binder: *R. R. Donnelley & Sons, Harrisonburg, VA*
Page Layout: *Jonathan B. Waugh*
Illustrations by: *Linda D. Waugh*

©1999 by Prentice-Hall Inc.
Pearson Education
Upper Saddle River, New Jersey   07458

Printed in the United States of America
10 9 8 7 6 5 4 3

ISBN 0-13-081427-X

Prentice-Hall International (UK) Limited, *London*
Prentice-Hall of Australia Pty. Limited, *Sydney*
Prentice-Hall Canada Inc., *Toronto*
Prentice-Hall Hispanoamericana, S.A., *Mexico*
Prentice-Hall of India Private Limited, *New Delhi*
Prentice-Hall of Japan, Inc., *Tokyo*
Prentice-Hall (Singapore) Asia Pte. Ltd., *Singapore*
Editora Prentice-Hall do Brasil, Ltda., *Rio de Janeiro*
Prentice-Hall, Inc., Upper Saddle River, New Jersey

CONTENTS

PREFACE

This text introduces ventilator waveforms. It is intended to serve as a compliment to a mechanical ventilation textbook and as a reference convenient to carry in the clinical environment.

It would be impractical and ponderous to attempt to include all possible examples of ventilator waveforms that could be seen in the clinical setting. The goal of this book is to impart an understanding of how waveforms are generated which will allow the practitioner to deduce the cause and implications of previously unseen as well as familiar waveforms. Understanding waveforms instead of memorizing many patterns aids in problem-solving and correction of abnormal conditions and prepares clinicians to adapt to future yet unknown modes of ventilation.

The rationale behind the format of this text was to provide a simple, portable reference and workbook that could be used at the bedside as well as the classroom. Descriptions and commentary were kept to a minimum to enhance clarity and readability. Ventilator waveform topics that are experimental, in limited use, or not considered mainstream were not included in keeping with this book's introductory theme.

The first chapter provides clean, easy to read conceptual illustrations to aid in comprehension. Examples of real waveforms are provided next to the conceptual renderings to allow the learner to become comfortable with viewing waveforms with normal artifact present. The following chapters utilize mostly real recordings of ventilator waveforms. Scalars and loops are discussed in the first two chapters. The third chapter provides side-by-side comparisons of the majority of current ventilator modes. Chapter four provides examples of common clinical findings and chapter five is devoted to neonatal waveforms. Several neonatal and adult case studies are provided in the appendix for practice.

CHAPTER 1
VENTILATOR GRAPHICS AND CLINICAL APPLICATIONS

BASIC CONCEPTS

Four basic parameters are most descriptive of mechanical ventilation: pressure, volume, flow, and time. Conventionally, these parameters are plotted against each other to reflect changes associated with changes in pathology. Normally, three graphs, called scalars comprising of flow vs. time, volume vs. time, and pressure vs. time are used. Other graphs such as flow-volume loop and pressure-volume loop provide quick information on certain changes in lung function. In order to be consistent in initial parameters the following example will serve as a baseline and a reference point to compare any variations in the settings or in lung functions.

CLINICAL EXAMPLE

The following example is designed to demonstrate to the reader how the computerized graphic system incorporated in the ventilators actually draws these waveforms based on the set parameters and calculated parameters. The example provides illustrations of effects of changes in ventilator modes on the tracings of pressure, volume, and flow plotted against time.

A post-open heart patient is brought in the intensive care unit and placed on a volume ventilator on the following parameters:

Tidal Volume (V_T)	750 mL or 0.75 L
Respiratory Frequency (f)	15 breaths/min or respiratory cycles/min
Inspiratory Flow Rate (V)	30 L/min
Airways Resistance (R_{AW})	10 cm H_2O/L/sec
Respiratory System Compliance (C_{RS})	0.05 L/cm H_2O or 50 mL/cm H_2O
Mode	Control

1

EFFECT OF SETTING CHANGES ON WAVEFORMS

Changes made on mechanical ventilator settings result in predictable changes in the graphics. Similarly, changes in the lung characteristics such as R_{AW} and C_{RS} can be recognized from specific variations in the waveforms. Figures 1-1, 1-2, and 1-3 demonstrate the effects of changes in parameters on the ventilator graphics.

Refer to Figures 1-1A and 1-1B and observe the effects of changing respiratory frequency on the cycle time (T_C), other parameters are unchanged. Figures 1-2A and 1-2B demonstrate the effect of changing inspiratory flow rate on the inspiratory time (T_I) and expiratory time (T_E). Notice in Figure 1-3 that the effects of increased airway resistance on the resistance pressure and the peak inspiratory pressure (PIP). Figure 1-4 depicts the effect of decreased C_{RS} on alveolar pressure and PIP.

INTERRELATIONSHIP BETWEEN THE CYCLE TIME AND THE RESPIRATORY RATE: (Figure 1-1) Cycle time strictly depends on the set respiratory rate. Figures 1-1A and 1-1B demonstrate the effects of changes in respiratory frequency on the flow vs. time scalar.

From the initial settings: $V_T = 750$ mL, f = 15 cycles/min, V = 30 L/min, the cycle time can be calculated,

$$T_C = \frac{60 \text{ sec/min}}{\text{frequency}} = \frac{60 \text{ sec/min}}{15 \text{ cycles/min}} = 4 \text{ sec.}$$

The cycle time consists of inspiratory and expiratory time. The inspiratory time is calculated from the delivered tidal volume and the inspiratory flow rate. In this case the inspiratory time is 1.5 seconds, thus the remaining time 2.5 seconds accounts for the expiratory time.

Figure 1-1A: If the respiratory rate is increased to 20 cycles/min, the cycle time decreases to 3 seconds and the expiratory time decreases to 1.5 seconds.

$$T_C = \frac{60 \text{ sec/min}}{\text{frequency}} = \frac{60 \text{ sec/min}}{20 \text{ cycles/min}} = 3 \text{ sec.}$$

Figure 1-1B: Observe the effect of changing the respiratory rate from 15/min to 12/min. Cycle time increases from 4 seconds to 5 seconds.

$$T_C = \frac{60 \text{ sec/min}}{\text{frequency}} = \frac{60 \text{ sec/min}}{12 \text{ cycles/min}} = 5 \text{ sec.}$$

Since the inspiratory time remains unchanged, the expiratory time increases from 2.5 seconds to 3.5 seconds (T_E = Tc - T_I = 5 sec - 1.5 sec = 3.5 sec).

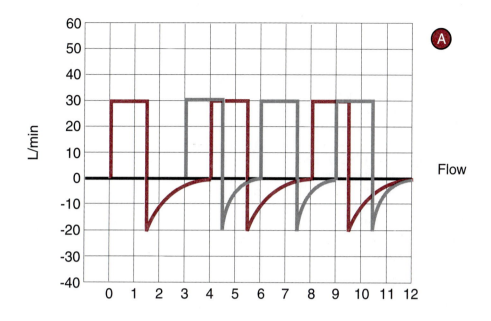

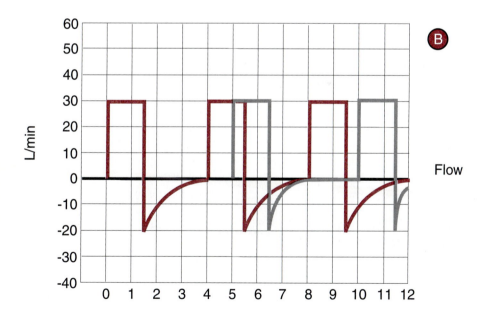

Figure 1-1A and 1-1B. The effects of changing respiratory frequency on the cycle time.

EFFECT OF FLOW RATE ON INSPIRATORY AND EXPIRATORY TIME:

(Figure 1-2) Increased inspiratory flow rate decreases inspiratory time and allows for a longer expiration time, conversely if the flow rate is decreased, the inspiratory time increases and the expiratory time decreases.

The inspiratory time can be calculated by dividing the delivered tidal volume by the inspiratory flow rate. For the initial settings, $V_T = 750$ mL, f = 15 cycles/min, V = 30 L/min, $T_C = 4$ sec, $T_I = 1.5$ seconds, $T_E = 2.5$ seconds, and inspiratory flow rate = 30 L/min = 30 L/60 sec = 0.5 L/sec = 500 mL/sec.

$$T_I = \frac{\text{tidal volume}}{\text{flow rate}}$$

$$T_I = \frac{\text{tidal volume}}{\text{flow rate}} = \frac{750 \text{ mL}}{500 \text{ mL/sec}} = 1.5 \text{ sec}$$

Figure 1-2A: The graphic indicates the effect of increasing flow rate from 30 L/min to 60 L/min. Notice that the inspiratory time decreased from 1.5 seconds to 0.75 seconds and the expiratory time increased from 2.5 seconds to 3.25 seconds. Recognize that the cycle time remained 4 seconds. If the flow rate is doubled from 30 L/min to 60 L/min, the inspiratory time decreases by half, from 1.5 seconds to 0.75 seconds, thus allowing for a longer expiratory time (3.25 seconds).

$$T_I = \frac{\text{tidal volume}}{\text{flow rate}} = \frac{750 \text{ mL}}{1000 \text{ mL/sec}} = 0.75 \text{ sec}$$

Figure 1-2B: If the inspiratory flow rate is decreased, the inspiratory time increases. This is shown in Figure 1-2B. The inspiratory flow rate is decreased from 30 L/min to 22.5 L/min (22.5 L/min = 22.5 L/60 sec = 0.375 L/sec = 375 mL/sec). The change in flow rate increases the inspiratory time from 1.5 seconds to 2.0 seconds which in turn decreases the expiratory time from 2.5 seconds to 2.0 seconds.

$$T_I = \frac{\text{tidal volume}}{\text{flow rate}} = \frac{750 \text{ mL}}{375 \text{ mL/sec}} = 2.0 \text{ sec}$$

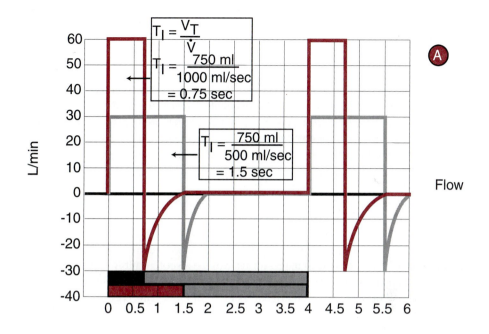

$$T_I = \frac{V_T}{\dot{V}}$$

$$T_I = \frac{750 \text{ ml}}{1000 \text{ ml/sec}} = 0.75 \text{ sec}$$

$$T_I = \frac{750 \text{ ml}}{500 \text{ ml/sec}} = 1.5 \text{ sec}$$

Flow

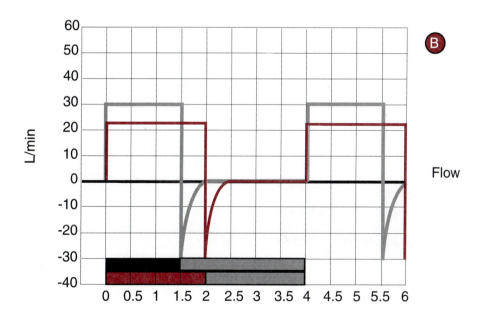

Flow

Figure 1-2A and 1-2B. Effect of changing inspiratory flow rate on inspiratory time and expiratory time.

EFFECT OF RESISTANCE AND COMPLIANCE CHANGES: Figures 1-3 and 1-4 demonstrate the effects of changes in airways resistance and decreased respiratory system compliance on the pressure/time scalar.

Pressures plotted on the pressure/time scalar are calculated from the known parameters of R_{AW}, C_{RS}, the inspiratory flow rate, and the delivered tidal volume. During an inspiration and expiration, the gas flow encounters resistance in the airways. The molecular frictional activity results in development of pressure. This pressure is equal to the product of R_{AW} and the gas flow rate. The pressure required to overcome R_{AW} as gas flows through the airways is the airway resistance pressure (P_{RAW}).

$$
\begin{aligned}
P_{RAW} \quad &= \quad \text{flow rate x } R_{AW} \\
&= \quad 0.5 \text{ L/sec x } 10 \text{ cm } H_2O/L/sec \\
&= \quad 5 \text{ cm } H_2O
\end{aligned}
$$

Once the gas molecules reach the alveolar region, the force required to deliver a given tidal volume to the lungs against the recoil force of the alveoli results in a pressure. This pressure is known as alveolar pressure (PA). Since this pressure is obtained from an inspiratory hold or plateau, it is referred to as $P_{plateau}$ or P_{static}. This pressure is calculated from the tidal volume and C_{RS}.

$$
P_{plateau} \quad = \quad \frac{\text{tidal volume}}{C_{RS}}
$$

Since the $V_T = 750$ mL and $C_{RS} = 0.05$ L/cm $H_2O = 50$ mL/cm H_2O

$$
P_{plateau} \quad = \quad \frac{750 \text{ mL}}{50 \text{ mL/cm } H_2O} \quad = 15 \text{ cm } H_2O
$$

Knowing the two pressures, P_{RAW} and $P_{plateau}$, the PIP can be obtained.

$$
\begin{aligned}
PIP \quad &= \quad P_{RAW} + P_{plateau} \\
&= \quad 5 \text{ cm } H_2O + 15 \text{ cm } H_2O \\
&= \quad 20 \text{ cm } H_2O
\end{aligned}
$$

Figure 1-3: Provides a graphical view of increased R_{AW} on the pressure/time scalar. Notice that as the R_{AW} increases the pressure required to overcome airway resistance increases as does the PIP. Initial parameters indicated a $P_{RAW} = 5$ cm H_2O, $P_{plateau} = 15$ cm H_2O and the PIP = 20 cm H_2O. If the airway resistance doubles due to increased secretions, bronchospasm or any other obstruction, the P_{RAW} increases to 10 cm H_2O and the PIP increases to 25 cm H_2O.

Figure 1-4: This figure demonstrates that as the lung compliance decreases the static or plateau pressure increases resulting in increased peak pressure. If the compliance decreases by half (25 ml/cm H_2O) the plateau pressure will increase to 30 cm H_2O and the PIP will increase to 35 cm H_2O.

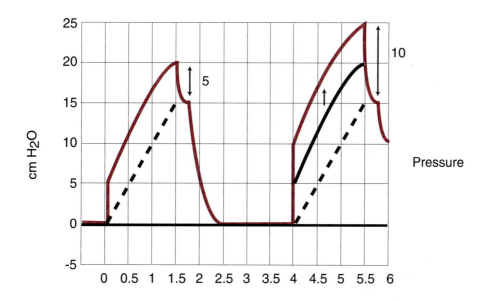

Figure 1-3. The effect of airways resistance on the pressure waveform.

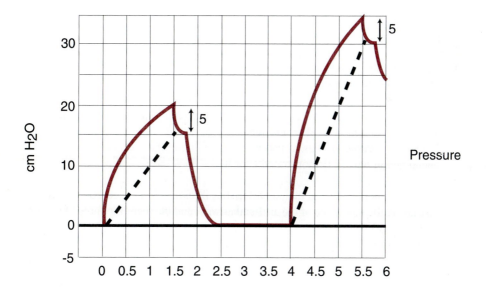

Figure 1-4. The effect of changing respiratory system compliance on the pressure waveform.

SCALARS

A mechanical breath in a graphical format can be viewed in stages, (Figure 1-5)
  A. Beginning of inspiration
  B. Inspiration
  C. End of inspiration
  D. Beginning of expiration
  E. Expiration
  F. End of expiration

Five stages of a mechanical breath are indicated below: (Figure 1-5)

A. *Beginning of inspiration* depends on the triggering mechanism. In the control mode or in a situation where the ventilator provides backup ventilation, the ventilator initiates mechanical breath on elapse of a predetermined time. This is termed as *time triggered breath*. In the assist mode or a Synchronized Intermittent Mandatory Ventilation (SIMV) mode, the mechanical breath is initiated by the patient's effort. This is termed as *patient triggered breath.*

B. During *inspiration* the mechanical breath is delivered and the flow, volume, and pressure characteristics of the breath depend on various factors such as, airway resistance, lung compliance, type and magnitude of the flow, and the tidal volume being delivered.

C. The clinicians determine the parameter responsible for *termination of inspiration* referred to as cycling mechanism. These mechanisms include volume cycling, pressure cycling, time cycling, and flow cycling.

D. Generally, during mechanical ventilation, when inspiration ends, the *expiratory phase begins* by opening the exhalation valve. However, in special situations, such as when the inspiratory pause or inflation hold controls are activated, the exhalation valve does not open even though inspiratory gas flow has stopped. The delivered volume is held inside the lungs to obtain static or plateau pressure. Expiration begins in this situation upon opening the exhalation valve. This phenomenon will be demonstrated later in the book.

E. *Exhalation* is passive and the characteristics of exhalation depend on the airways resistance, the resistance of the artificial airway, and the recoiling force of the lung (compliance).

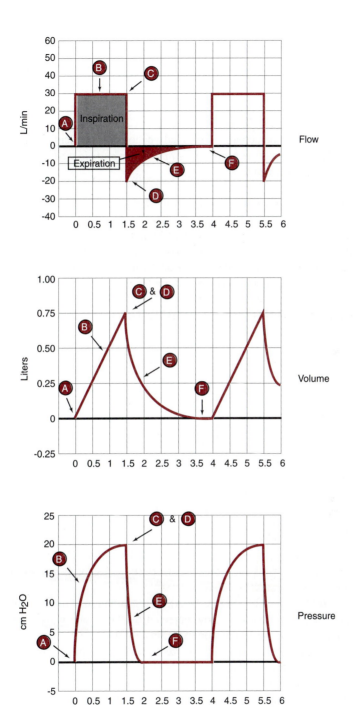

Figure 1-5. Components of the breath cycle.

MODES OF VENTILATION AND CORRESPONDING SCALARS

Figures 1-6 to 1-11 demonstrate the six (6) modes commonly employed in mechanical ventilation. Each set of scalars is shown in two formats--a clean graphic form drawn using the parameters given in the example and an actual waveform generated from a mechanical ventilator graphic module. The reader should compare these two sets of graphics to appreciate the actual and cleaned versions of the identical waveforms. *In later chapters, only the actual graphics will be shown and cleaned ones will be shown only when deemed necessary.*

Figure 1-6:   Control mode
Figure 1-7:   Assist mode
Figure 1-8:   Synchronized Intermittent Mandatory Ventilation (SIMV)
Figure 1-9:   SIMV with Pressure Support ventilation (PSV)
Figure 1-10:   SIMV with PSV and Positive End expiratory Pressure (PEEP)
Figure 1-11:   Pressure Control Ventilation (PCV)

CONTROL MODE VENTILATION: (FIGURE 1-6)

Notice the following:
a.   On each graph the inspiratory time and expiratory times correspond to termination of inspiration and expiration respectively.
b.   *A negative deflection of the tracing is observed on the flow/time curve only.* This is because the flow transducer measures inspiratory flow (positive deflection), as well as, expiratory flow (negative flow).
c.   The square flow tracing indicates a constant flow ventilator.
d.   Since the flow is constant, the volume delivery is rectilinear (straight line increase).
e.   The initial rise in the pressure to 5 cm H_2O corresponds to the pressure required to overcome airway resistance (P_{raw}). Beyond this point the increase in pressure depends on the lung compliance and the volume delivered up to that point. Near the end of the delivery of tidal volume, the pressure contour has flattened due to delivery of volume in almost filled lungs.
f.   At the end of inspiration (1.5 sec) the flow delivery stops, all the tidal volume is delivered, and the peak inspiratory pressure (P_{peak}) has been reached.

FLOW VS. TIME SCALAR: (Figure 1-6A) At the initiation of mechanical ventilation the ventilator delivers a constant flow depicted by the square wave form. The flow instantaneously reaches the set level of 30 L/min and continues for 1.5 seconds ($T_I = V_T/$ flow). At this time the flow decreases to zero and expiration begins. The transducer reports expiratory flow on the negative side of the scale. This flow reaches it's maximum level immediately and tapers up to zero during exhalation. The next inspiration does not begin until the set cycle time (Tc = 60 sec/f) of 4 seconds has elapsed and the tracing continues.

VOLUME VS. TIME SCALAR: (Figure 1-6B) The electronics mathematically performs integration of the flow/time tracing to determine the volume/time tracing. Since the flow rate is constant, the volume is delivered in fixed increments per unit time resulting in a straight line tracing. The delivery of volume is terminated when the set tidal volume of 750 mL is delivered. The exhalation begins and volume decays to the baseline. The next volume delivery begins when the cycle time elapses.

PRESSURE VS. TIME SCALAR: (Figure 1-6C) At the beginning of inspiration the gas flow experiences the frictional resistance of the airways. Throughout the flow of the gas molecules within the airways molecular bombardment on each other and on the surrounding walls of the airways generates a pressure. The abrupt rise of 5 cm H_2O pressure represents the pressure resulting from the airway resistance (P_{RAW} = flow x R_{AW}). After overcoming the frictional resistance, the gas now flows into the alveoli and encounters elastic resistance. Since the inspiratory phase does not terminate until the set tidal volume is delivered, the respiratory compliance promotes a gradual increase in pressure strictly dependent on the volume delivered and the lung compliance ($P_{plateau}$ = V_T/C_{RS}). In this case the plateau pressure of 15 cm H_2O and the P_{RAW} of 5 cm H_2O account for the peak inspiratory pressure of 20 cm H_2O. At the end of inspiration (1.5 sec) the pressure quickly decreases to the baseline (zero pressure). The next tracing appears after 4 seconds (T_C).

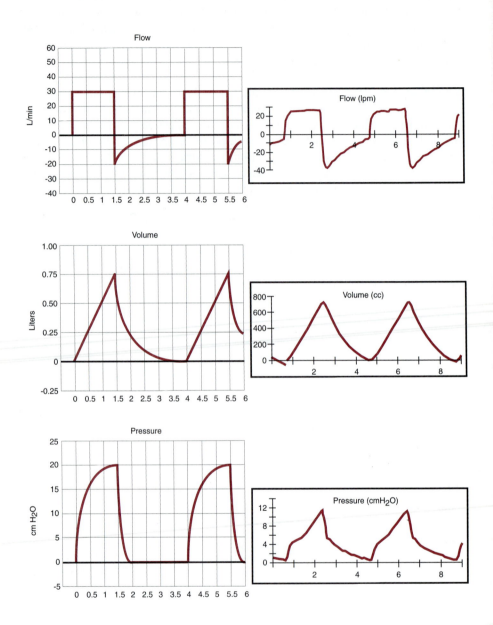

Figure 1-6A, 1-6B, and 1-6C. Volume-targeted control ventilation mode.

ASSIST MODE VENTILATION: (FIGURE 1-7) Parameter changes: The inspiratory flow rate was increased to 60 L/min and the ventilator was switched to deliver assisted breaths at the rate of 12 breaths/min. However, the patient reset his rate to 20 breaths/min. Notice that these parameter adjustments also changed other calculated parameters.

$$T_c \text{ decreased to } \frac{60 \text{ sec/min}}{20 \text{ cycles/min}} \quad = \quad 3 \text{ seconds}$$

T_I decreased to 0.75 seconds as a result of increased flow rate from 30 L/min to 60 L/min

$$T_{I=} \quad \frac{750 \text{ ml}}{1000 \text{ ml/sec}} \quad = \quad 0.75 \text{ sec.}$$

P_{raw} also increased due to increased flow rate
$$P_{raw} = \text{Flow Rate x } R_{aw}$$
$$= \frac{1 \text{ L}}{\text{sec}} \text{ x } \frac{10 \text{ cm H}_2\text{O}}{\text{L/sec}}$$
$$= 10 \text{ cm H}_2\text{O}$$

And the PIP increases proportionately,
$$PIP = P_{raw} + P_{static} = 10 + 15 \text{ (cm H}_2\text{O)}$$
$$= 25 \text{ cm H}_2\text{O}$$

Notice the following:
a. With increased flow rate the inspiratory time shortened and allowed the patient to increase the respiratory rate to 20/min. The flow rate instantaneously reaches to 60 L/min and stays constant for 0.75 sec.
b. A small negative deflection on the pressure/time graph indicates patient triggering characteristic of all assisted breaths.
c. The initial rise of 10 cm H_2O pressure is due to the pressure required to overcome airways resistance. Consequently, the PIP reaches 25 cm H_2O.

FLOW VS. TIME SCALAR: (Figure 1-7A) Similar to the control ventilation the ventilator delivers a constant flow throughout the inspiratory phase as shown by the square wave tracing. Since the flow rate was increased to 60 L/min, flow is maintained at 60 L/min for the duration of the inspiratory time (0.75 seconds). Concurrently, the set tidal volume is delivered and the flow drops to zero and expiration begins. As exhalation proceeds the flow gradually returns to the baseline. The next inspiration begins after 3 seconds.

VOLUME VS. TIME SCALAR: (Figure 1-7B) Similar to the volume/time tracing in the controlled mode, volume delivery is a straight line increase. The delivery of volume is terminated when the set tidal volume of 750 mL is delivered. The exhalation begins and volume decays to the baseline. The next volume delivery begins when the cycle time elapses.

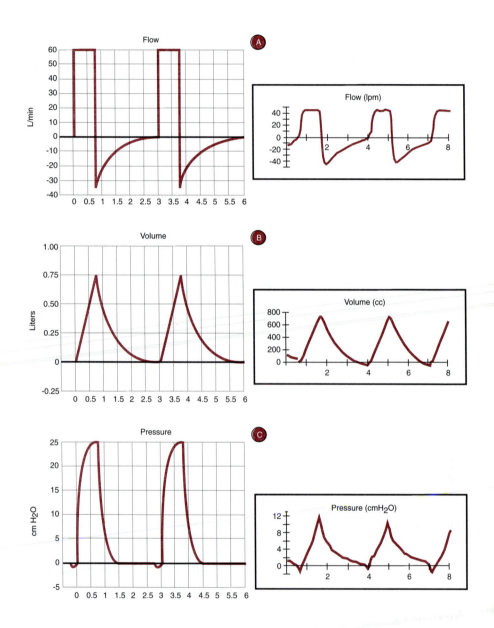

Figure 1-7A, 1-7B, and 1-7C. Volume-targeted assist-control ventilation.

PRESSURE VS. TIME SCALAR: (Figure 1-7C) Compared to the pressure/time graph in the controlled mode certain differences are obvious. A small negative deflection indicates that the breath was initiated by the patient (patient-triggering), thus called assisted breath. The first 10 cm H_2O pressure is attributed to the pressure due to the airways resistance (P_{RAW} = flow x R_{AW}). Since lung compliance did not change the pressure required to deliver the tidal volume into the lungs is the same (15 H_2O). As a result the total peak inspiratory pressure reaches 25 H_2O in 0.75 seconds (inspiratory time). At this time the inspiration ends since the tidal volume is delivered (volume cycling). The exhalation valve opens and the pressure quickly decreases to the baseline.

SIMV: (FIGURE 1-8) Parameter changes: On the assisted ventilation at a rate of 20/min the patient was hyperventilating. It was decided to place the patient on an SIMV mode with a rate of 12 breaths /minute. This change resulted in an increase in the total rate to 36 breaths/minute indicating that between two mechanical breaths the patient was taking two spontaneous breaths of 150 mL tidal volume.

Notice the following:
a. Between two mechanical breaths the inspiratory flow tracing on spontaneous breaths is on the positive side of the graph and during expiratory phase the flow is registered below the baseline.
b. Spontaneous volume reaches 150 mL.
c. Unlike flow and volume, the inspiratory pressure is traced on the negative side of the baseline and exhalation shows a positive side tracing.
d. The beginning of inspiration, inspiration, termination of inspiration, and end of expiration on all breaths, mechanical as well as spontaneous, coincide on the time scale.

FLOW VS. TIME SCALAR: (Figure 1-8A) Observe that two spontaneous breaths occur in between two mechanical breaths. The mechanical breath has the same characteristics as in the assisted ventilation (Figure 1-2). For the spontaneous cycles, inspiratory flow is shown as a positive deflection and the expiratory flow as a negative contour. Since the SIMV rate is set at 12 /min, the mechanical cycle time is set at 5 seconds. Every five seconds the ventilator delivers a mechanical breath.

VOLUME VS. TIME SCALAR: (Figure 1-8B) The location where spontaneous breaths occur should coincide with the flow/time events. The volume delivered during spontaneous breath is only 150 mL where the volume curve reaches the peak. Again, the characteristics of the mechanical breaths are identical to those in the assisted ventilation (Figure 1-2).

PRESSURE VS. TIME SCALAR: (Figure 1-8C) Notice that the spontaneous breaths are represented by a negative deflection during inspiration and a positive deflection during exhalation. Also, the mechanical breaths are patient triggered as shown by a small negative deflection before the mechanical breath is initiated.

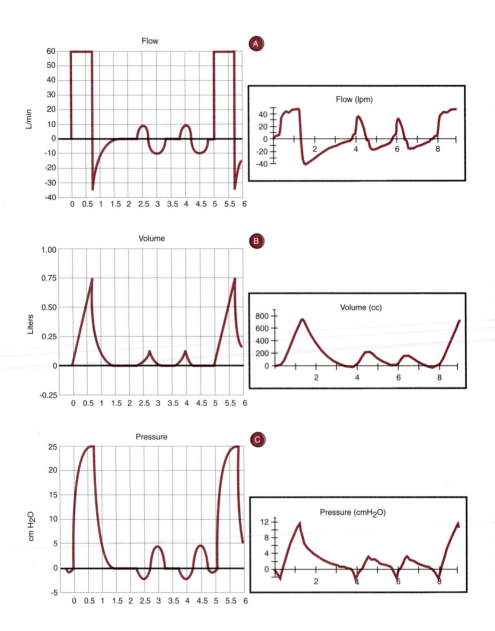

Figure 1-8A, 1-8B, and 1-8C. Synchonized Intermittent Mandatory Ventilation waveforms.

SIMV WITH PRESSURE SUPPORT VENTILATION: (FIGURE 1-9) Parameter changes: Since the spontaneous tidal volume was very small, a 10 cm H_2O Pressure Support was initiated. This manipulation increased the spontaneous tidal volume from 150 mL to 350 mL allowing the patient to decrease his respiratory rate from 36/min to 24/min indicating that the patient was interposing one spontaneous breath in between two mechanical breaths.

Notice the following:
a. On the flow/time scalar the pressure supported breath delivered a decreasing flow and terminated inspiration when the flow reached a certain level (flow cycling).
b. The volume delivery shows that during the spontaneous component of breathing a tidal volume of 350 mL is delivered.
c. Pressure supported breaths are delivered to maintain set pressure (10 cm H_2O in this case) throughout the inspiratory phase. The pressure decays during expiratory phase to the baseline. Also, observe that all breaths are patient triggered confirmed by the small negative deflection to the beginning of inspiration on the pressure/time scalar.

FLOW VS. TIME SCALAR: (Figure 1-9A) Notice the pressure supported breath is interposed between two mechanical breaths. The most striking characteristic of the pressure supported breath is its flow delivery. During inspiratory phase the flow tapers from its peak level. A pressure supported breath, generally, terminates inspiration when the inspiratory flow decreases to a system specific flow (usually 25% of the peak flow). Thus a pressure supported breath can be termed as a flow cycled breath.

VOLUME VS. TIME SCALAR: (Figure 1-9B) As a result of a pressure supported breath the spontaneous volume increased from 150 mL to 350 mL and the spontaneous ventilatory rate decreased. The patient is now initiating only one breath between two mechanical cycles.

PRESSURE VS. TIME SCALAR: (Figure 1-9C) Observe that the pressure is maintained to 10 cm H_2O throughout the inspiratory phase. Also notice that the spontaneous as well as the mechanical breaths are patient triggered as revealed by the negative deflections on the pressure/time waveform.

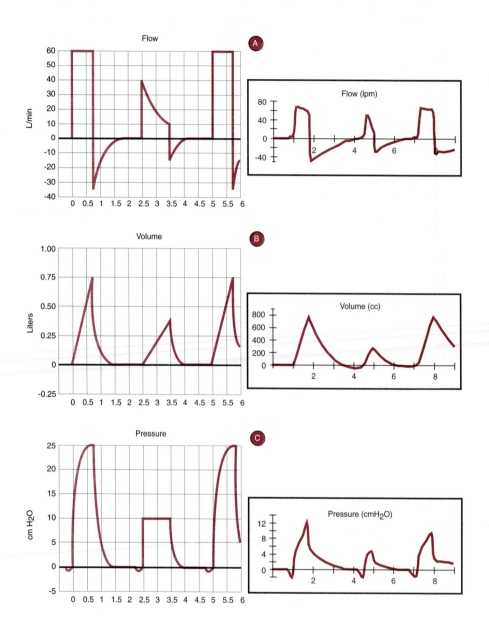

Figure 1-9A, 1-9B, and 1-9C. Synchonized Intermittent Mandatory Ventilation with Pressure Support Ventilation waveforms.

SIMV WITH PSV AND POSITIVE END EXPIRATORY PRESSURE:

(Figure 1-10) Parameter changes: Blood gas analysis indicated that the patient's ventilation was adequate, however, the oxygenation status was not acceptable. The patient showed a PaO_2 of 43 mm Hg on an F_IO_2 of 0.9. It was decided to initiate Positive End Expiratory Pressure (PEEP) to improve oxygenation. PEEP level was gradually increased and titrated with pulse oximetry (SpO_2). At a PEEP level of 15 cm H_2O the SpO_2 increased to 90%.

Notice the following:
a. Initiation of PEEP elevates the baseline on the pressure/time graph from zero to 15 cm H_2O resulting in the elevation of the peak pressure (PIP) from 25 cm H_2O to 40 cm H_2O.
b. On end of exhalation the airway pressure decreases to the new baseline of 15 cm H_2O.
c. On flow/time and volume/time tracing the baseline remains at the same level before instituting PEEP.

FLOW VS. TIME: (Figure 1-10A) Addition of PEEP does not change the flow pattern from the previous settings (Figure 1-9A).

VOLUME VS. TIME: (Figure 1-10B) The volume/time curve remains unchanged.

PRESSURE VS. TIME: (Figure 1-10C) Observe the baseline is elevated from zero to 15 cm H_2O. This resulted in the increase of the PIP from 25 cm H_2O to 40 cm H_2O.

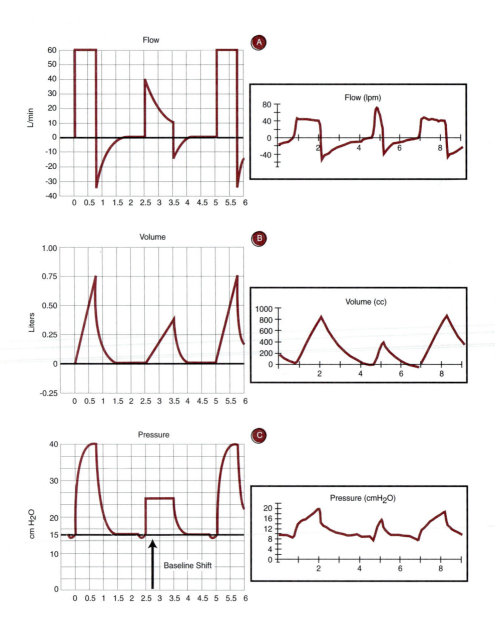

Figure 1-10A, 1-10B, and 1-10C. SIMV with PSV and PEEP.

PRESSURE CONTROL VENTILATION (PCV): (Figure 1-11) Parameter changes: The patient continued to deteriorate. The PIP gradually increased to 55 H_2O. It was decided to switch the patient from volume ventilation to pressure ventilation mode. The patient was sedated and the ventilator was adjusted to deliver Pressure Controlled Ventilation (PCV) at a level of 30 cm H_2O and at a respiratory rate of 15 breaths /min. The inspiratory time was set to 1.5 seconds and a backup rate at 12/min.

Notice the following:
a. The ventilator terminates inspiration when a preset time has elapsed (1.5 seconds in this case).
b. On the flow/time scalar the flow decreases to zero before the inspiration ends. The pressure stays at the set pressure throughout the inspiratory time.

FLOW VS. TIME: (Figure 1-11A) Since the pressure control mode is time cycled mode, the inspiratory flow continues to taper down throughout inspiratory phase and may reach to zero flow at or before the inspiratory time (1.5 seconds) elapses.

VOLUME VS. TIME: (Figure 1-11B) The delivered volume depends on the lung characteristics. The volume delivery is terminated at the end of inspiratory phase.

PRESSURE VS. TIME: (Figure 1-11C) Observe the baseline returns to zero since the PEEP was eliminated. The pressure is maintained at 30 cm H_2O during the inspiratory phase (1.5 seconds).

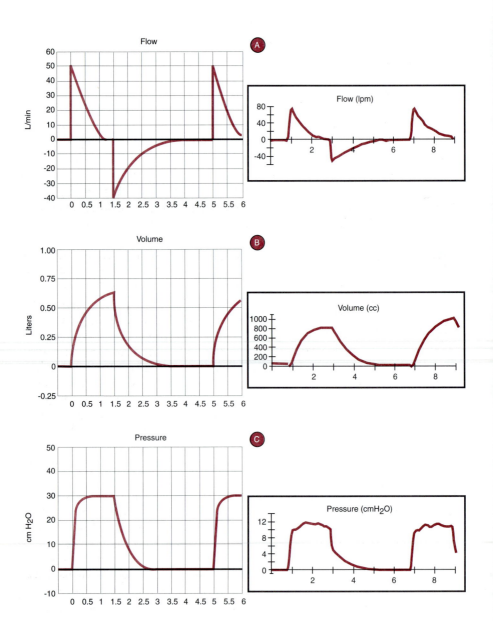

Figure 1-11A, 1-11B, and 1-11C. Pressure Control Ventilation.

CHAPTER 2
PRESSURE-VOLUME AND FLOW-VOLUME LOOPS

I.   Introduction
II.   Pressure-Volume Loops
III.   Work-of-Breathing
IV.   Flow-Volume Loops
V.   Interpretation of Loops

Pressure-volume (P-V) and flow-volume (F-V) loops are typically studied after becoming familiar with pressure, flow, and volume scalars. As with the scalars, information can be obtained from both numeric values and the shape of the waveforms. A loop is actually an inspiratory and expiratory curve connected together. It is common for clinicians to initially have difficulty with the fact that loops do not express units of time. The progression of a breath can be followed from beginning to end but without any reference to how much time has passed.

It is helpful to have in mind normal patterns, values, and conventions when evaluating P-V and F-V loops. The scale of the axes must be set so that the loops are displayed appropriately for analysis. For example, the P-V loop allows for quickly determining at a glance if a patient's dynamic compliance is abnormal by looking at the slope or pitch of the loop. A loop with normal compliance is conventionally displayed with a slope that is roughly at a 45 degree angle to horizontal. A normal dynamic compliance for a ventilator patient ranges 50-80 ml/cm H_2O[1] so the axes should be set so that a compliance value in the middle of that range (65 ml/cm H_2O) would be at about a 45 degree angle. In some instances it is helpful to scale the axes without regard for convention so that the screen displays as much of the loop as possible to better see details. Afterwards, return the axes scale to a conventional setting so that others can easily monitor patients' graphics even from a distance as they move about a unit or ward. P-V loops in this chapter do not necessarily conform to the 45 degree convention for normal compliance in order to magnify details and display a larger complete graphic.

Most readers may be familiar with F-V loops from pulmonary function studies but it is important to note that there is no convention for how the inspiratory and expiratory portions of the F-V loops are oriented with respect to horizontal axis. Traditionally, a pulmonary function report displays F-V loops with the inspiratory curve below the horizontal axis and the expiratory curve above the axis. Ventilator graphics displays may show this orientation or the reverse, depending on the brand of equipment. One common source of confusion associated with loop evaluation results from changing more than one ventilator or patient variable at a time. It is helpful to make incremental changes when using ventilatory waveforms to guide fine-tuning of the ventilator to the patient. For example, when trying to assess if a bronchodilator drug had a beneficial effect by comparing changes in the loops before and after treatment, changing the mode of ventilation between measurements may obscure or counterfeit improvements from the drug.

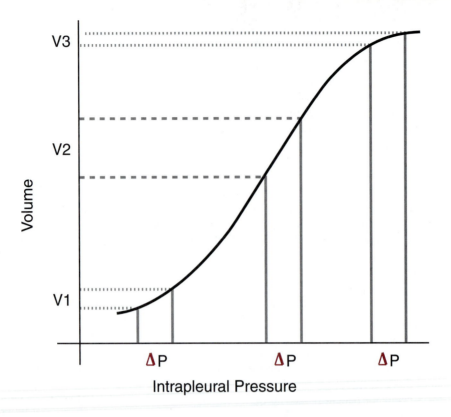

Figure 2-1. Volume as a function of position on the total lung compliance curve.

Compliance is the term commonly used in pulmonary physiology to describe the change in lung volume in relation to the change in intrapleural pressure. There are several specific variations of the term compliance used to discuss ventilatory conditions. The compliance curve produced by slowly inflating a patient's lungs with positive pressure might look similar to the one in Figure 2-1. The largest volume is obtained at the steepest portion of the curve, the middle. The baseline for tidal breathing is normally positioned in this same region allowing for spontaneous ventilation at the most efficient portion of the curve. When a pulmonary disorder such as atelectasis or air-trapping significantly increases or decreases the baseline for tidal breathing, ventilatory efficiency decreases. This results in decreased dynamic and static respiratory system compliances and distortion of the P-V loop in particular.

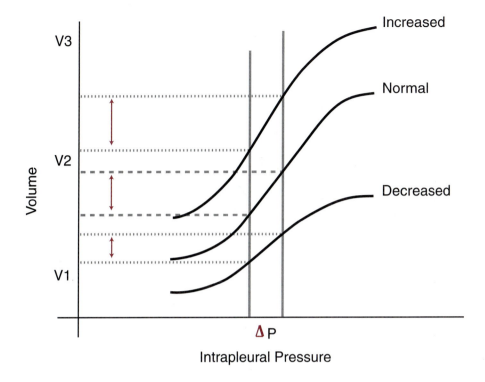

Figure 2-2. Shifts the lung compliance curve from pulmonary disorders yield different tidal volumes.

Not only are pulmonary disorders able to shift the tidal breathing origin to some abnormally high or low point on the total lung compliance curve but they can change the shape of the entire curve. Imagine inflating a patient's lungs very slowly so that airways resistance would be almost nonexistent while recording the inspiratory pressure-volume curve. The same pressure change applied to the middle portions of such curves with different slopes would produce different volumes (Figure 2-2).

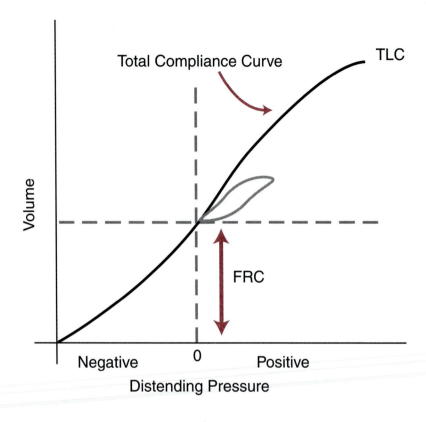

Figure 2-3. The tidal breath in relation to the total lung compliance curve.

A positive pressure tidal breath placed on the total compliance curve might look like the gray loop in Figure 2-3. Functional residual capacity (FRC) is an important term to understand when discussing relationships in ventilation and respiratory mechanics. The point of zero airway pressure indicates the balance between the lungs' tendency to recoil and the chest wall's tendency to expand outward. The volume of gas in the lungs at this balancing point is the FRC.

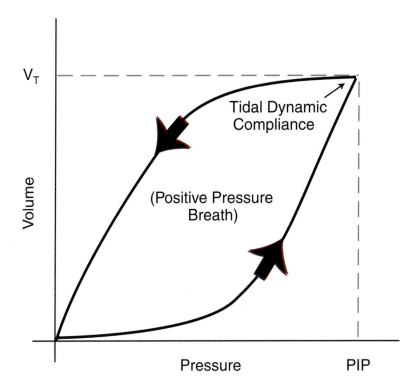

Figure 2-4. Components and labels of a positive pressure breath P-V loop.

Intubated patients are artificially ventilated by positive pressure breaths. When pressure (horizontal axis) and volume (vertical axis) changes are plotted against each other, a loop such as the one in Figure 2-4 is generated. Conceptual renderings of P-V loops are often elliptical or "football shaped" but such a symmetric pattern is not seen in reality. The breath begins in the lower left corner of the graph following the counterclock wise path indicated by the red arrows, finally ending at the lower left corner. The upper right corner of the loop marks the end of inspiration and the beginning of expiration. This point of maximal pressure and volume represents the dynamic compliance (change in volume divided by change in pressure) of the respiratory system for that breath. Note that the loop begins at zero pressure, indicating there is no positive pressure applied to the baseline (PEEP).

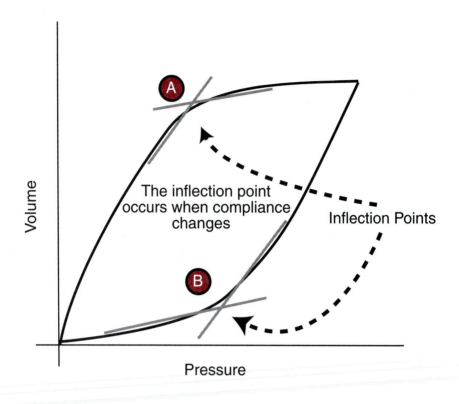

Figure 2-5. Inspiratory and expiratory inflection points of a positive pressure breath.

Changes in respiratory compliance can be detected in the P-V loop by noting shifts in the slope of the line. The point of change in the slope of a line is called the inflection point. The loop in Figure 2-5 has two inflection points, one during the expiratory phase (A) and one during the inspiratory phase (B). Every loop has at least two inflection points but some have more. If the inflection point is difficult to determine, it often helps to draw lines along the portions of the inspiratory and expiratory curves that are nearly straight as in Figure 2-5. The inflection point will be adjacent to the point of intersection for the two drawn lines. These inflection points are thought to represent sudden alveolar recruitment during inspiration and derecruitment of alveoli during expiration. Lung protective protocols often suggest setting PEEP with these in mind to minimize lung stress. Among clinicians the inspiratory inflection point is often referred to as the *inspiratory knee*.

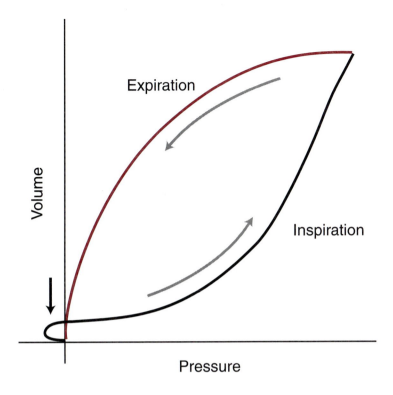

Figure 2-6. Assisted positive pressure ventilator breath.

A positive pressure ventilator breath produces a P-V loop similar to the examples in Figures 2-4 and 2-6. Figure 2-4 would represent what is termed a control breath, meaning it is triggered solely by the timing mechanism of the ventilator without any regard to whatever spontaneous efforts the patient may have. Figure 2-6 represents a ventilator breath that is triggered by a spontaneous patient respiratory effort. There are many variations of positive pressure breaths but they will be dealt with in Chapter Three. As previously described, inspiration (represented by the black line segment) starts at the intersection of the axes in the lower left corner of the graph. The small bulge into the negative side of the pressure axis (see black arrow) represents the patient's effort to begin inspiration. At the point the ventilator senses the patient's effort and starts a machine breath, the line shifts rightward into the positive side of the pressure axis. Expiration starts at point of highest volume and pressure and is represented by the red line segment. Except for the initial patient effort, both inspiratory and expiratory phases of the ventilator breath occur on the positive pressure side of the pressure axis.

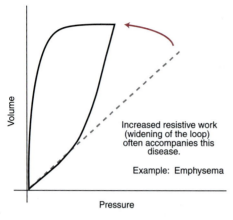

Increased resistive work (widening of the loop) often accompanies this disease.

Example: Emphysema

Figure 2-7. Increased respiratory system compliance.

Recall that the convention for displaying normal dynamic compliance is to have the point of end inspiration displayed so that a line traced to the beginning point of inspiration would be approximately 45 degrees to the horizontal axis (represented by the dotted line in Figure 2-7). An increase in respiratory system compliance causes a shift to the left of the 45 degree line.

Patients with emphysema typically have wide P-V loops with increased compliance (Figure 2-7). The widening of the loop is caused by airway resistance which is described later in this chapter. Changes in compliance are not necessarily accompanied by changes in resistance. Increases in compliance often are gradual except in circumstances such as the administration of surfactant therapy.

A decrease in compliance causes a rightward shift in the loop as indicated in Figure 2-8. Variations of this pattern are typically seen in the later stages of acute respiratory distress syndrome (ARDS). Decreases in compliance can occur gradually as in the progression of a pulmonary disease or suddenly such as when large airways become plugged by mucous or by the endotracheal tube advancing into the right mainstem bronchus.

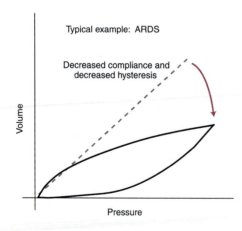

Typical example: ARDS

Decreased compliance and decreased hysteresis

Figure 2-8. Decreased respiratory system compliance.

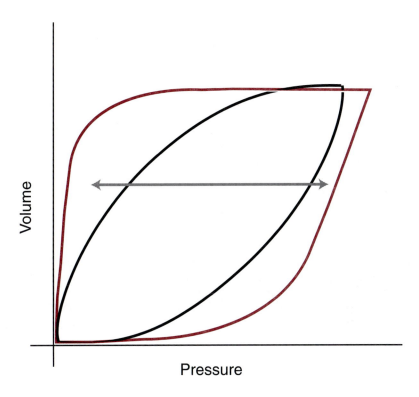

Figure 2-9. Increased airways resistance produces exaggerated P-V loop hysteresis.

Changes in airways resistance cause the area of the P-V loop and its horizontal distance to increase (Figure 2-9). These changes result from hysteresis, a lag in the volume change in relation to the rate of pressure change due to increased airways resistance. Notice that the widened red loop has a greater peak pressure and a slightly lower peak volume than the black loop. The ventilator must apply more pressure to move less volume which indicates a decrease in ventilatory efficiency. The slight rightward shift indicates the resistance is creating a decreased compliance effect. The normal airways resistance range for an intubated patient (up to 5 cm $H_2O/L/sec$) is slightly higher than for a nonintubated patient.[2] It is difficult for even experienced clinicians to identify increased airways resistance simply by looking at a P-V loop unless the hysteresis is profound or two loops are superimposed for comparison. F-V loops are more commonly used for bronchodilator benefit testing on ventilator patients. However, F-V loops obtained during volume-targeted ventilation do not show inspiratory-only increases in airways resistance well so it is a good habit to review both F-V and P-V loops for changes in airways resistance.

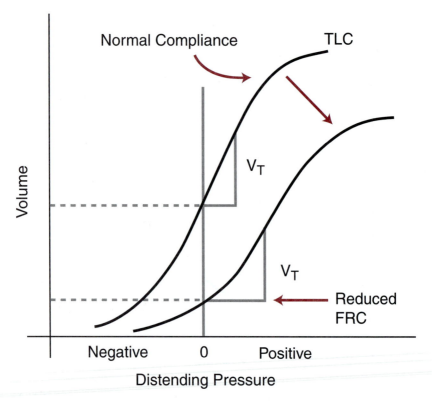

Figure 2-10. Pressure-volume relationship determines work-of-breathing.

The compliance curves in Figure 2-10 are similar to those in Figures 2-1 and 2-2 but show the zero pressure reference point. The importance of FRC to ventilatory efficiency becomes clear when volumes generated for a given pressure change at different points on the total lung compliance curve are compared. The same volume is moved on the normal and low compliance curves but the pressure required to do so is nearly doubled on the curve with decreased compliance. The amount of pressure required to move a particular volume is related to what is termed the "work" done during each breath. The work done during a breath on the rightmost curve is greater due to both the decreased compliance (slope of the curve) and the decreased FRC (position of the zero pressure point on the curve). The work-of-breathing (WOB) can be measured several ways but discussion will only involve the method involving ventilatory graphics also termed "mechanical WOB."

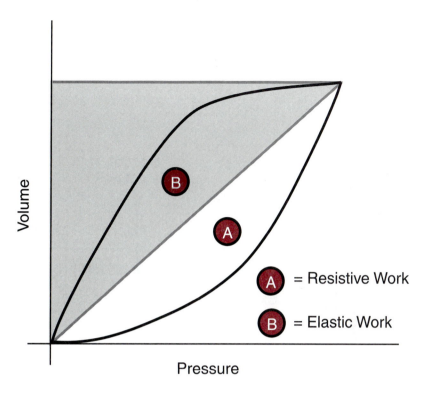

Figure 2-11. The WOB components for a positive pressure breath.

The WOB can be done by the patient, the ventilator, or be shared by both. The WOB components for a positive pressure ventilator breath are labeled in Figure 2-11. The unshaded portion of the P-V loop marked "A" represents the WOB due to overcoming airways resistance. The shaded area labeled "B" represents the WOB required to stretch the elastic lung tissue during inspiration. Together, A and B represent the total mechanical work done during the breath. The WOB is typically expressed as an integral, where WOB equals the area under the changing pressure curve as volume moves from zero to its peak at end inspiration. This may be more clear if you turn the P-V loop 90 degrees to the left so that volume is on the x-axis. The greater the area comprised by A and B, the greater the WOB. Most ventilator graphic displays show only the mechanical work measured at the airway opening (the endotracheal tube connector). This method is reliably accurate only if the patient is not contributing any ventilatory efforts (essentially paralyzed). Patient contributions to WOB during mechanical breaths can be indirectly measured by plotting esophageal pressures.

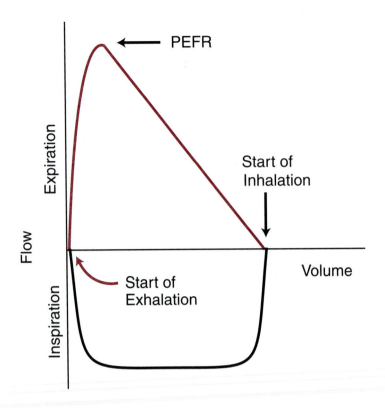

Figure 2-12. Components and labels of a normal positive pressure breath F-V loop.

The F-V loop recorded during mechanical ventilation looks similar to the F-V loop reported in PFT studies but the two differ in that the mechanical breaths do not represent maximal spontaneous efforts as do the PFT breaths. In Figure 2-12 the vertical axis represents flow rate (liters per second) and the horizontal axis represents volume (usually in liters for adults). The inspiratory portion of the F-V loop (black) is below the horizontal axis and the expiratory portion (red) is above it. Recall that this orientation may be reversed depending on the brand of equipment. Normally, the transition from inspiration to expiration and back again occurs where the loop crosses the horizontal axis when the flow rate is momentarily zero. The shape of the inspiratory curve will reflect the flow pattern set on the ventilator, which is a constant flow rate or square wave in this case. The highest point above the x-axis represents the peak or maximal expiratory flow rate (PEFR) during a passive exhalation. The shape of this passive expiratory curve will be influenced by anything that may cause airway obstruction.

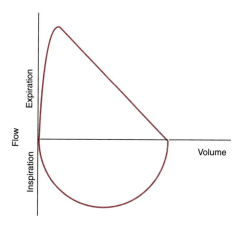

Figure 2-13. Conceptual sinusoidal flow pattern for a positive pressure ventilator breath.

The rendering in Figure 2-13 represents a perfect sinusoidal (sine) pattern that looks similar in shape to those seen in PFT studies. Note that the orientation of the inspiratory and expiratory portions of the loop in Figure 2-14 are opposite of Figure 2-13. The shape can be altered by patient variations, ventilator settings, circuit conditions, and the way in which the breath is generated by the ventilator. Although the peak flow rates are different for the two breaths in Figure 2-14 the shapes are similar. Exhalation is passive but because this particular ventilator did not deliver the same volume at both flow rate settings, the expiratory flow pattern is slightly altered.

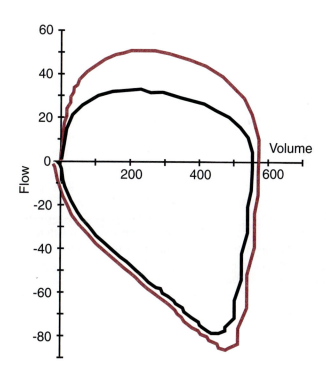

Figure 2-14. Recorded sinusoidal flow pattern at two flow rate settings.

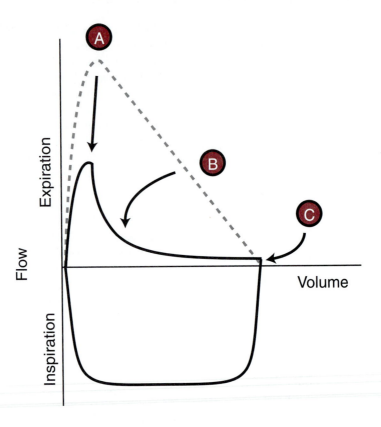

Figure 2-15. Signs of airwary obstruction in the F-V loop.

Airways obstruction can cause several changes in the F-V loop depending on the type and severity. The gray dashed line in Figure 2-15 represents the normal expiratory flow pattern for the example patient and the arrows indicate possible deviations from this normal pattern due to obstruction. Most types of significant airways obstruction will reduce the maximal expiratory flow rate (item A in Figure 2-15). Medium and small airways obstruction also tend to cause the descending segment of the expiratory curve to take on a curvilinear shape (item B in Figure 2-15) which is often termed "scooping" in the clinical setting. Air-trapping may occur if expiratory time is insufficient or the smaller airways collapse prematurely due to abnormal anatomic changes. Air-trapping is identified in Figure 2-15 item C, the expiratory portion of the loop not returning to baseline (zero flow rate) before the start of the next breath.

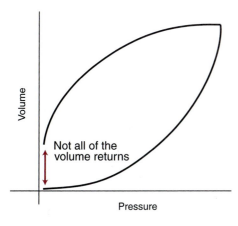

Figure 2-16. Volume loss present in the P-V loop.

Volume loss during a breath can be detected in both loop and scalar formats. Volume loss due to some type of leak appears on a waveform as an expiratory volume smaller than the inspiratory volume. The volume lost to leaks that occur downstream from the flow transducer used to generate the loop graphics (on the patient side of the transducer) will appear as part of the inspiratory volume. The lost volume is not returned through the flow transducer so the loop does not close. The gap indicated by the red arrow in Figure 2-16 indicates a partial loss of volume during expiration. Likewise the gap identified by the arrow in Figure 2-17 indicates a volume loss. Possible sources of such leaks include endotracheal tube cuff leaks, bronchopleural fistula, and air leaks through chest tubes. An inspiratory volume that is less than the set volume but has an equivalent expiratory volume would not be due to such a leak. Equally diminished inspiratory and expiratory volumes could be produced by a leak in the ventilator circuit between the flow transducer and the ventilator.

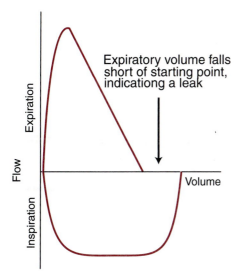

Figure 2-17. Volume loss present in the F-V loop.

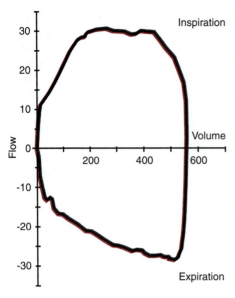

Figure 2-18. Spontaneous breath F-V loop.

Loop waveforms of spontaneous breaths differ in a few ways from positive pressure ventilator breaths. F-V loops are similar except for the inspiratory portion of the loop. The inspiratory curve of a spontaneous breath is rounded, much like a ventilator breath set to the sine wave pattern (Figure 2-14). The principal difference is lower peak flow rate typically observed with spontaneous breaths (Figure 2-18). Expiration is passive so the shape is consistently a descending ramp-like pattern for both spontaneous and ventilator breaths.

The differences between spontaneous and ventilator breath P-V loops are more obvious. Spontaneous breaths are generated as negative pressure is created in the chest. This causes a leftward bulge of the P-V loop into the negative side of the pressure axis (Figure 2-19). The loop is traced in a clockwise fashion. Exhalation occurs on the positive side of the pressure axis, mirroring the change to positive pressure in the chest and airways during expiration.

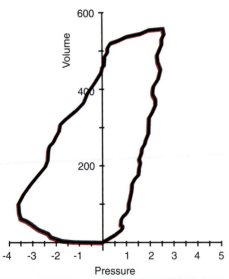

Figure 2-19. Spontaneous breath P-V loop.

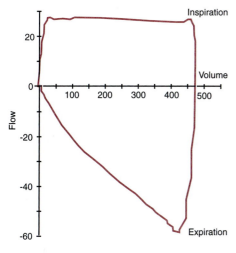

Figure 2-20. F-V loop from a square wave flow pattern positive pressure ventilator breath.

A ventilator breath with a constant flow pattern, also called a "square wave" pattern is displayed in Figure 2-20. The flow rate remains the same throughout most of inspiration. This in turn produces a fairly constant volume delivery. Although this pattern is not used as often as a descending flow pattern, it is helpful for detecting abnormalities in the P-V loop precisely because flow and volume delivery are constant. Note in Figure 2-21 that the P-V loop has not been scaled to display the slope of a normal dynamic compliance line at roughly a 45 degree angle to the horizontal axis. Recall that a normal dynamic compliance for a ventilator breath ranges from 50-80 ml/cm H_2O. The volume change of 550 ml divided by the pressure change of 13 cm H_2O dynamic yields a dynamic compliance of 42 ml/cm H_2O. The slope of this loop would actually fall below the 45 degree convention. Note the absence of any negative pressure deflection in the P-V loop, thus indicating this is probably a control mode breath.

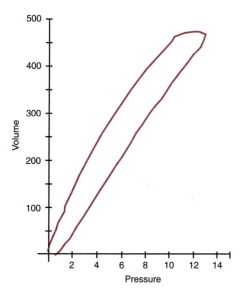

Figure 2-21. P-V loop from a square wave flow pattern positive pressure ventilator breath.

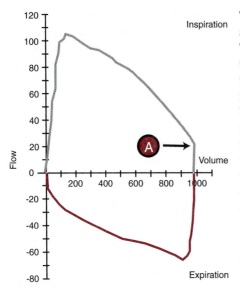

Figure 2-22. A F-V loop from a PSV breath.

The PSV breath shown in Figure 2-22 is another type of positive pressure breath. The F-V loop appears at first glance to be two opposing expiratory curves joined together. The inspiratory phase is shown in gray and the expiratory in red. A PSV breath has a characteristic that can be mistaken for an abnormal clinical condition previously described as auto-PEEP (Figure 2-15). Note the abrupt change in the slope of the inspiratory curve indicated by point "A" on the inspiratory curve. This sudden drop towards the horizontal axis at the <u>end of inspiration</u> is due to the ventilator cycling from inspiration to expiration when gas is still flowing to the patient. Auto-PEEP is identified as a sudden return to baseline at the <u>end of exhalation</u>, beginning of inspiration. Therefore, when inspiratory and expiratory flow patterns look similar, it is especially important to orient yourself as to how inspiration and expiration are displayed on the F-V loop graph.

The P-V loop in Figure 2-23 shows the same PSV breath and color-coding as in Figure 2-22. Note that the inspiratory and expiratory lines cross each other at about +2 cm H_2O instead of next to the volume axis (as in Figure 2-6). This is due in this case to the patient making a vigorous attempt to inspire during the PSV breath. The inspiratory curve is not smoothly curved because of the patient effort.

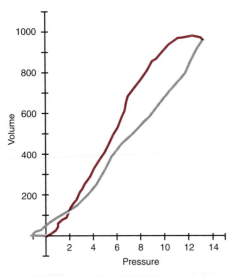

Figure 2-23. A P-V loop from a PSV breath.

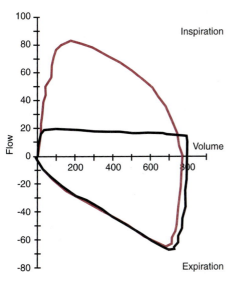

Figure 2-24. F-V loops from a volume-targeted breath (black) and pressure-targeted breath (red).

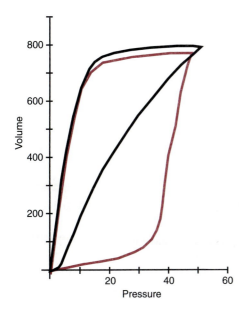

Figure 2-25. P-V loops from a volume-targeted breath (black) and pressure-targeted breath (red).

A comparison of volume and pressure-targeted ventilator breaths is shown in Figures 2-24 and 2-25. In both figures, the volume-targeted breath is black and the pressure-targeted breath is red. The volume-targeted breath has a constant flow pattern which makes it easy to distinguish the inspiratory and expiratory segments of the F-V loop. The pressure-targeted F-V loop is similar to the PSV loop except that it does not have the sudden drop in flow to the horizontal axis at the end of the inspiratory period.

The set pressure for the pressure-targeted breath is similar to the peak pressure observed with the volume-targeted breath (Figure 2-25). Notice that the horizontal diameter and hysteresis are much greater for the pressure-targeted breath. This is not surprising since the flow rate is much higher for this mode throughout inspiration. Keep in mind that resistance and compliance for the respiratory system remain the same for both breath types in this example.

It would be inaccurate to attribute the increased hysteresis seen in the pressure-targeted breath as increased airways resistance. That is why it would be inappropriate to change from volume to pressure-targeted ventilation mode or vice-versa between a pre and post-bronchodilator comparison or while assessing the effect of adjusting other ventilator control variables to fine-tune ventilation.

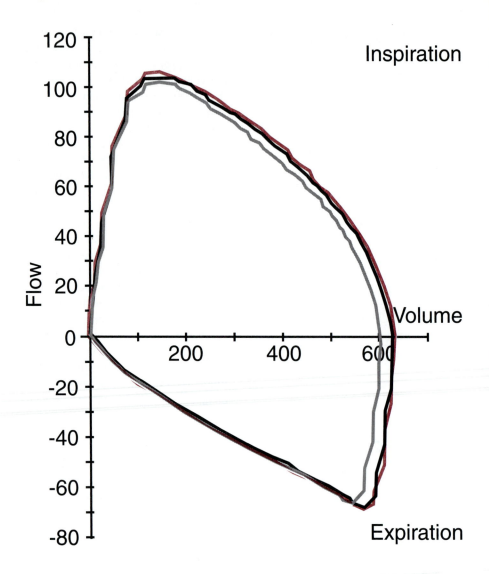

Figure 2-26. PCV breaths with long, short, and no inspiratory pauses.

The F-V loop in Figure 2-26 is enlarged primarily to show the difference in volume between three pressure-targeted breaths with varying inspiratory pauses. The term "inspiratory pause" is somewhat confusing in this case because although the pressure is held constant creating a plateau, volume is allowed to change. The gray loop represents no inspiratory pause, the black loop has short pause, and the red loop has the longest pause. In patients that have a wide range of time constants, such as with ARDS, pneumonia, etc., a pressure plateau during a PCV breath can allow for additional volume delivery without increasing pressure. Inspiratory plateaus are also thought to improve distribution of ventilation.

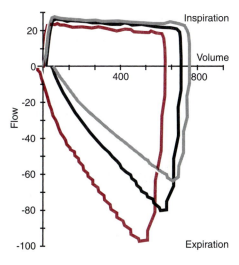

Figure 2-27. The effect of compliance changes on positive pressure breath F-V loops.

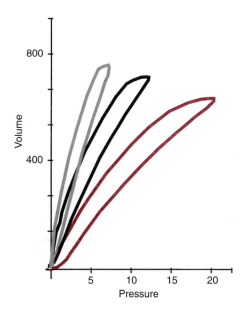

Figure 2-28. The effect of compliance changes on positive pressure breath P-V loops.

Changes in respiratory compliance are best seen in P-V loops but there are predictable changes that occur in F-V loops as well. A constant flow mode is used in Figure 2-27 to best isolate the effect of changing compliance. Red represents the lowest compliance, black is a moderate compliance, and gray is the highest compliance. The tidal volumes increase as compliance increases. Inspiratory peak flows remain similar but the expiratory peak flow rates decrease as compliance increases. This pattern is related to the concept of elastic WOB described in Figure 2-11. Work is done during inspiration to stretch the elastic tissue in the lung and thorax. The stored force is released during expiration. An increase in compliance is associated with a decrease in the elastic recoil of the lungs. The less elastic recoil present, the less stored energy to be released during exhalation. That is why the peak expiratory flow rates are less as compliance increases.

The P-V graph in Figure 2-28 shows three different respiratory compliances with the same airways resistance value. The gray loop represents increased compliance, the black loop represents normal compliance, and the red loop represents decreased compliance. Decreasing compliance is sometimes referred to as a "right-shift" in the P-V loop. Although increased hysteresis can accompany a decrease in compliance they are not linked, as seen in this figure.

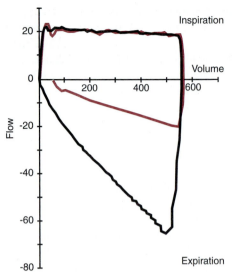

Figure 2-29. A F-V loop with normal inspiratory and increased expiratory airways resistance.

Increased airways resistance can occur during inspiration, expiration, or both. The F-V loop in Figure 2-29 contrasts two constant flow breaths, one with normal airways resistance (black) and the other with increased expiratory airways resistance (red). Notice the decreased peak expiratory flow rate. No scooping is observed, which is consistent with obstruction in the large airways. The shortened return of the red loop indicates a small leak.

The F-V loop for the same breath in Figure 2-30 dramatically show the effect of increased expiratory resistance. Note that the inspiratory curves are essentially the same, only the expiratory curves differ. Causes of increased resistance during expiration-only include diseases that cause early small airways collapse such as emphysema, bronchomalacia, and the patient biting the endotracheal tube during the expiratory phase.

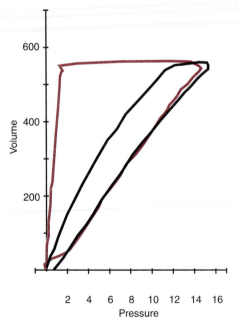

Figure 2-30. A P-V loop with normal inspiratory and increased expiratory airways resistance.

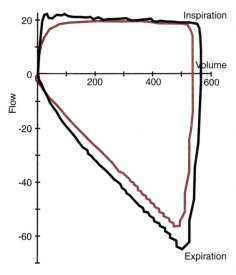

Figure 2-31. A F-V loop with increased inspiratory and normal expiratory airways resistance.

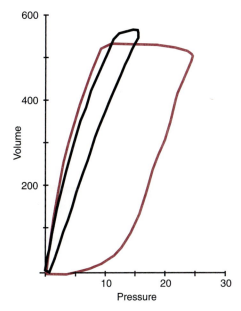

Figure 2-32. A P-V loop with increased inspiratory and normal expiratory airways resistance.

The normal loop is in black and the loop with increased inspiratory resistance is red. The effect of increased inspiratory resistance on the F-V loop in Figure 2-31 is minimal. That is because the driving force of the ventilator is sufficient to overcome the increased resistance. Slightly less volume was delivered so the peak expiratory flow rate was correspondingly less.

The P-V loop in Figure 2-32 impressively shows the increase in inspiratory resistance. The expiratory curves are similar except the volume of the normal curve is slightly greater as observed in the F-V loop. The tidal volume is affected more by inspiratory resistance than expiratory resistance. In ventilator patients there are few causes of increased resistance during inspiration-only because of the airway-splinting effect of positive pressure ventilation and the endotracheal tube. Examples include the patient biting the endotracheal during inspiration or the rare occurrence of a pedunculated mass (growth attached by a stalk) intermittently blocking an airway, producing a ball-valve effect.

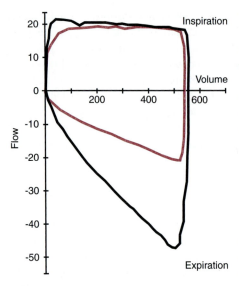

Figure 2-33. A F-V loop with both increased inspiratory and expiratory airways resistance.

The two constant flow loops in Figure 2-33 show the combined effects of those in Figures 2-29 and 2-31. The red loop is a result of increases in resistance throughout the entire ventilator breath. Other than a slight rounding of the square inspiratory flow pattern, the only changes from the normal black loop occur in the expiratory portion.

It is clear that the red P-V loop in Figure 2-34 that corresponds to the red F-V loop in Figure 2-33 reveals more deviations from the normal. Though the increased hysteresis is obvious, without the normal curve present it would be difficult to determine whether it was due to increased resistance during inspiration, expiration, or both. Also, the greater the resistance, the more that volume is decreased from the set value.

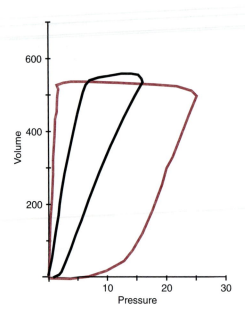

Figure 2-34. A P-V loop with both increased inspiratory and expiratory airways resistance.

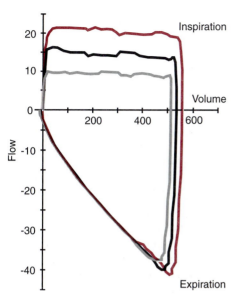

Figure 2-35. F-V loops for volume-targeted positive pressure breaths at three different peak flow rates.

Adjusting peak flow rate in volume-targeted ventilation can produce a variety of changes in ventilator waveforms. It is clear that the flow rate is changing from 20 to 15 to 10 L/min (red, black, and gray respectively). In this particular ventilator, decreasing the peak flow rate resulted in a related decreases in tidal volume. This in turn yielded decreases in expiratory peak flow rate. This fluctuation in the delivered volume in spite of not changing the volume control setting may or may not occur, depending on the brand and model of the ventilator in use.

Flow rate impacts how much resistance develops as a breath is delivered. The progression of P-V loops in Figure 2-36 shows how loop hysteresis decreases as flow rate decreases. With all other variables remaining the same, the decrease in hysteresis that accompanies decreases in flow rate therefore indicates a drop in resistance (P-V loop colors correspond to the F-V loop breaths in Figure 2-35). Therefore, when the flow rate is adjusted to optimize ventilation, such as increasing peak flow rate to extend expiratory time for a patient with airways obstruction, the resulting change in the loop graphic should not be interpreted as a change in the patient's airways.

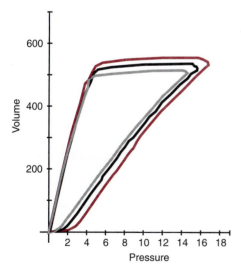

Figure 2-36. P-V loops for volume-targeted positive pressure breaths at three different peak flow rates.

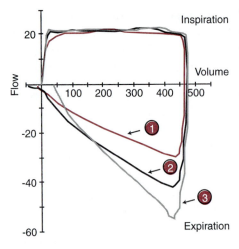

Figure 2-37. F-V loops for volume-targeted breaths with different airways resistances at a compliance of 50 ml/cm H_2O.

The graphic in Figure 2-37 is an example of changing airways resistance with a compliance near the low end of the normal range. If loop 1 represents the condition with the highest resistance, would loop 2 or 3 represent normal? Actually, all three loops represent conditions of abnormally high airways resistance though loop 3 is only mildly abnormal. Although a single F-V loop can often be used to detect obstruction due to increased airways resistance it is more useful when loops can be compared over time or before and after a change or therapy. Notice that as peak expiratory flow decreases, there is no "scooping." This suggests that the site of obstruction is in the large airways.

The P-V loops in Figure 2-38 clearly show the increase in hysteresis that accompanies increased airways resistance. Comparing loops 1 and 2 to the condition with the least resistance, loop 3, shows resistance is present on both inspiration and expiration. Waveform monitors that allow loops to be stored in memory for later comparison are very helpful but small printers can also be used to create printouts for comparisons. Waveform hardcopy from printers is also useful for giving report to colleagues or later creating a case study on an interesting patient.

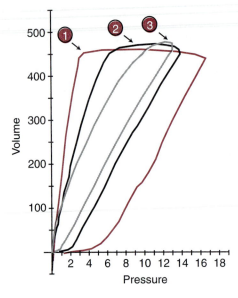

Figure 2-38. P-V loops for volume-targeted breaths with different airways resistances at a compliance of 50 ml/cm H_2O.

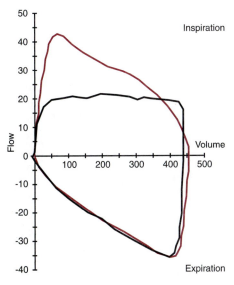

Figure 2-39. F-V loops for pressure and volume-targeted breaths with increased airways resistance and decreased compliance.

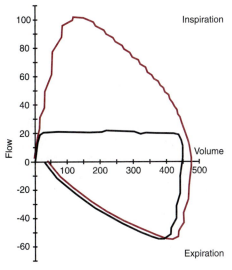

Figure 2-40. F-V loops for pressure and volume-targeted breaths with normal airways resistance and decreased compliance.

The F-V loops in Figure 2-39 contrast a pressure-targeted (red) and a volume-targeted (black) breath in the undesirable situation of both increased airways resistance (20 cm H_2O/L/second) and decreased compliance (20 mL/cm H_2O). If the increased resistance is due to bronchospasm and a bronchodilator is administered, the loops in Figure 2-40 result. The resistance decreased to a normal value 2 cm H_2O/L/second) and the compliance remained the same.

Notice that the constant flow inspiratory portion of the volume-targeted breath's F-V loop remains the same but the maximum expiratory flow rate increased. This is expected because the flow rate and pattern are actively controlled in the volume mode whereas expiration is passive and flow rate is influenced by changes in the patient's lungs.

The F-V loop for the pressure-targeted breath in Figure 2-39 undergoes changes in both the inspiratory and expiratory segments. Flow rates increase in both phases of the breath and the volume increases slightly, comparing Figures 2-39 and 2-40. This is another way of viewing the effects of changing airway resistance pressure described in Chapter One.

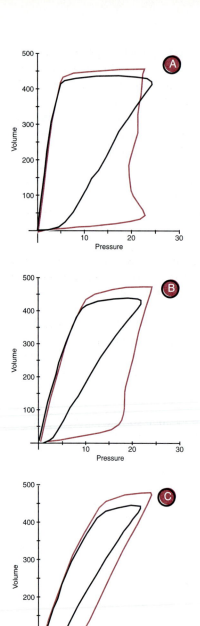

The P-V loops associated with the breaths in Figures 2-39 and 2-40 are depicted in Figure 2-41. The progression from "A" to "C" shows the effect of decreasing airways resistance while maintain a low compliance of 20 ml/cm H_2O. More changes occur in the P-V loop when resistance changes so three steps of change are displayed in Figure 2-41. The volume-targeted breaths in A, B, and C (black) have P-V loops of similar shape except for the hysteresis. The horizontal aspect of the loops appears to shrink proportionately. The pressure-targeted breaths exhibit a less proportional response to changing resistance. Under the highest resistance conditions, the pressure-targeted loop (red) shows an initial bulge that exceeds the pressure at the point of peak volume. As resistance decreases from A to B, the protrusion lessens. From B to C the primary change is a relatively proportional decrease in the width of the loop. This pattern makes sense when the F-V loops are examined. Recall that the pressure-targeted loop in Figure 2-39 had a much higher flow rate during inspiration, especially at the beginning. Under conditions of normal resistance and compliance the P-V loop of a pressure-targeted breath is very similar to a volume-targeted breath. However, high airways resistance exaggerates the effect of the higher flow pattern for the pressure breath such that the pressure curve begins to follow the pattern of the flow curve.

Figure 2-41. P-V loops alterations during changing resistance.

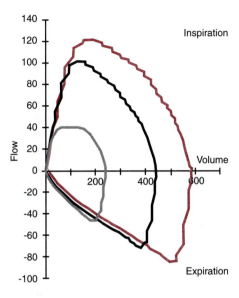

Figure 2-42. The effect of changing pressure levels on F-V loops in PCV mode.

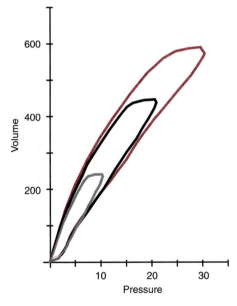

Figure 2-43. The effect of changing pressure levels on P-V loops in PCV mode.

The effect of changing set pressure levels for pressure-targeted breaths produces a predictable pattern as seen in Figure 2-42. As pressure increases, volume increases. Notice the brief plateau in inspiratory flow rate for the loop with the lowest pressure (gray). A typical ventilator in PCV mode has a high initial flow rate to quickly raise the airway pressure to the set pressure and maintain it for the set inspiratory time. Therefore peak flow rate is influenced by the conditions of the patient's lungs. Likewise, since only one control variable can be controlled at a time (pressure in this case), volume also changes as flow rate changes.

The P-V loops in Figure 2-43 reveal that resistance and compliance remain fairly constant in this example as peak pressure increases. These P-V loops of pressure-targeted breaths would appear very similar to those of volume-targeted breaths if under the same conditions of low airways resistance. There is no one characteristic shape for a pressure-targeted breath P-V loop. It depends greatly on the conditions in the patient's lungs. The important thing is to understand how the loop shape will change as resistance and compliance change, whether due to changes in anatomy or other ventilator variables.

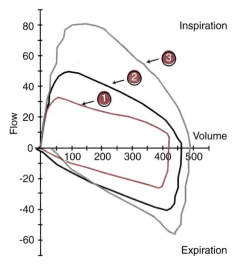

Figure 2-44. The effect of changing airways resistance with normal compliance on F-V loops during PCV.

Final examples of how pressure-targeted F-V and P-V loops can change as a result of different resistance and compliance combinations are given in Figures 2-44 and 2-45. In these examples, compliance is normal for each breath as resistance decreases from loop 1 to loop 3. Notice the sign of air-trapping in loop 1. The F-V loop is constrained to a near rectangular shape as the set pressure is quickly reached due to the increased airways resistance. As resistance decreases, the loops take on more of the typical decelerating ramp pattern.

The P-V loops in Figure 2-45 show a similar pattern as Figure 2-41 but in a superimposed format. In this case, a greater increase in volume is seen as resistance is withdrawn because the compliance is greater than in Figure 2-41. It would be difficult to gauge the degree of resistance if loop 1 or 2 were displayed alone. The goal is to learn how to identify abnormal shapes and compare two or more loops to each other, not to make absolute determinations of the degree of abnormality. Again, the goal is not to memorize shapes but to understand how they are created. This is essential for interpreting the causes of the countless abnormal shapes that are seen in the clinical setting.

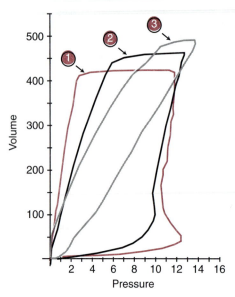

Figure 2-45. The effect of changing airways resistance with normal compliance on P-V loops during PCV.

REFERENCES

1.   Tobin MJ (ed.): Principles and practice of mechanical ventilation, New York, 1994, McGraw-Hill, Inc.

2.   Broseghini C, Brandolese R, Poggi R, et. al.: Respiratory resistance and intrinsic positive end-expiratory pressure (PEEP) in patients with the adult respiratory distress syndrome (ARDS). Eur Respir J 1988;1:726-31.

CHAPTER 3
WAVEFORMS FOR COMMON VENTILATOR MODES

I.   Volume-Targeted Scalars
             Control, Assist, SIMV
II.   Pressure-Targeted Scalars
             Control, Assist, SIMV
III.   Spontaneous Scalars
             CPAP, PSV, CPAP with PSV
IV.   Combination Modes: Volume-Targeted Scalars
             SIMV with CPAP, SIMV with PSV, SIMV with CPAP and PSV
V.   Combination Modes: Pressure-Targeted Scalars
             SIMV with CPAP, SIMV with PSV, SIMV with CPAP and PSV
VI.   Volume-Targeted Pressure-Volume (P-V) and Flow-Volume (F-V) Loops
             Control, Assist, SIMV
VII.   Pressure-Targeted P-V and F-V Loops
             Control, Assist, SIMV
VIII. Spontaneous P-V and F-V Loops
             CPAP, PSV, CPAP with PSV
IX.   Combination Modes: Volume-Targeted P-V and F-V Loops
             SIMV with CPAP, SIMV with PSV, SIMV with CPAP and PSV
X.   Combination Modes: Pressure-Targeted P-V and F-V Loops
             SIMV with CPAP, SIMV with PSV, SIMV with CPAP and PSV

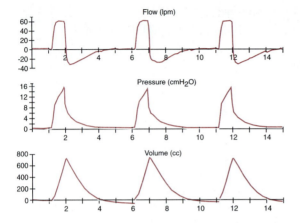

Figure 3-1. Volume-targeted control ventilation.

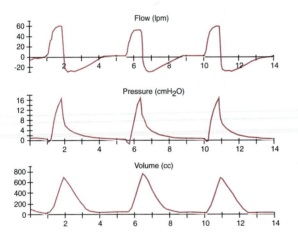

Figure 3-2. Volume-targeted assist/control ventilation.

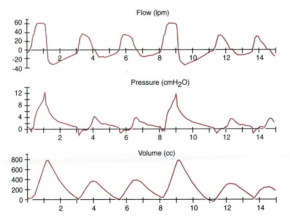

Figure 3-3. Volume-targeted SIMV.

VOLUME-TARGETED VENTILATION SCALARS

VOLUME-TARGETED CONTROL VENTILATION: *Time triggered, flow limited, volume cycled ventilation.* Each breath is a ventilator breath. Patient triggering does not occur.
WAVEFORM CHARACTERISTICS: (Figure 3-1) **Flow/time** scalar indicates a square flow (constant flow). **Pressure/ time** waveform confirms time triggering as each breath is delivered at a fixed time interval (pre-selected rate on the machine). **Volume/time** scalar displays a linear increase in the volume delivery. The ventilator breath terminates inspiration when the preset tidal volume is delivered (volume cycling).

VOLUME-TARGETED ASSIST/CONTROL VENTILATION: *Patient triggered, flow limited, and volume-cycled.* Each ventilator breath is triggered by the patient. In the event of apnea, control breaths are delivered at a preset backup rate.
WAVEFORM CHARACTERISTICS: (Figure 3-2) **Flow/time** scalar indicates similar pattern as in the control ventilation with a constant inspiratory flow. **Pressure/time** waveform differentiates a control breath from an assisted breath by the small negative deflection prior to the delivery of the mechanical breath. The assisted breath can be either pressure or flow triggered. **The pressure/time tracing is the only scalar that identifies a patient (pressure) triggered breath.** In case of apnea a backup rate is set by the clinician. **Volume/time** scalar shows a fixed tidal volume being delivered. Regardless of rapid triggering rate by the patient the delivered tidal volume does not change.

VOLUME-TARGETED SIMV: Spontaneous breaths are interposed between mechanical breaths. Pre-selected mechanical breaths (set by the rate control) are delivered at preset tidal volumes. The patient is allowed to breath spontaneously in between the mechanical breaths.
WAVEFORM CHARACTERISTICS: (Figure 3-3) **Flow/time** graphics demonstrate mechanical breaths delivered at a constant flow rate. The spontaneous breaths are indicated by lower flows and non-constant flow patterns. There are two spontaneous breaths interposed between each mechanical breaths. **Pressure/time** scalar demonstrates two low pressure tracings between two higher pressures associated with the mechanical breaths. Observe that the mechanical breaths are assisted and synchronized breaths as demonstrated by a small negative deflection before the breath is delivered. The negative portion of the spontaneous breath reflects inspiration, whereas the positive part of the tracing is associated with expiration. **Volume/time** tracing displays smaller volumes delivered during spontaneous component of the SIMV cycle.

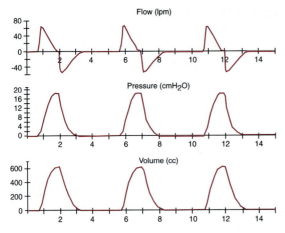

Figure 3-4. Pressure-targeted control ventilation.

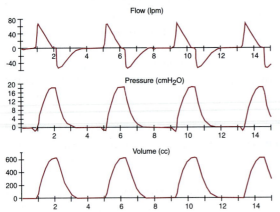

Figure 3-5. Pressure-targeted assist/control ventilation.

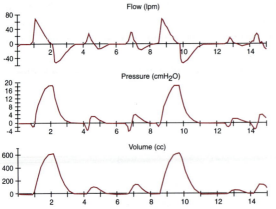

Figure 3-6. Pressure-targeted SIMV.

PRESSURE-TARGETED VENTILATION SCALARS

PRESSURE-TARGETED CONTROL VENTILATION: *Time triggered, pressure limited, time cycled ventilation.* Each breath is a controlled mechanical breath. This mode can be employed for ventilating patients in acute respiratory failure, especially in situations where the lung compliance is decreased.
WAVEFORM CHARACTERISTICS: (Figure 3-4) **Flow/time** scalar identifies a pressure controlled breath. Each breath is delivered at a fixed time interval. The flow descends throughout inspiration. The inspiratory phase terminates when the preset inspiratory time elapses (time cycling). **Pressure/time** scalar shows a sustained pressure (plateau) at the preset pressure level. **Volume/time** tracing is similar to the pressure/time curve in that the volume plateau is commonly observed. The volume decline occurs upon opening of the exhalation valve when the preset inspiratory time has elapsed.

PRESSURE-TARGETED ASSIST/CONTROL VENTILATION: Patient triggered, pressure limited, time cycled ventilation. Each breath is a ventilator breath triggered by the patient (pressure or flow triggered). In the event of apnea, control breaths are delivered at a preset backup rate.
WAVEFORM CHARACTERISTICS: (Figure 3-5) **Flow/time** tracing is consistent with that during control ventilation. The flow gradually tapers down to the baseline during the inspiratory time. Occasionally, the flow falls to the baseline before the inspiratory time has elapsed . However, in such a case, the exhalation valve does not open and a zero flow state is observed. **Pressure/time** scalar shows a small negative deflection prior to delivery of a mechanical breath consistent with the triggering effort made by the patient. Each breath is patient triggered. The peak pressure plateaus until the inspiratory time is over. **Volume/time** tracing is similar to the control breath.

PRESSURE-TARGETED SIMV: All mechanical breaths are delivered as pre-selected pressure control breaths (assisted) with interposed spontaneous breaths. Each breath is patient triggered breath, unless the patient becomes apneic, at which time the controlled breaths are delivered at the pre-selected backup rate.
WAVEFORM CHARACTERISTICS: (Figure 3-6) **Flow/time** tracing shows the pressure control breaths (assisted) with characteristic descending flow pattern. Notice that exhalation does not begin until the set inspiratory time has elapsed. **Pressure/time** pattern shows a pressure plateau during mechanical breaths. The spontaneous breaths are identified from the inspiratory phase below the baseline and the expiratory phase above the baseline. **Volume/time** waveform indicates an increased delivery of volume, a volume plateau, and a decline to the baseline during mechanical breaths. Note the smaller spontaneous breaths.

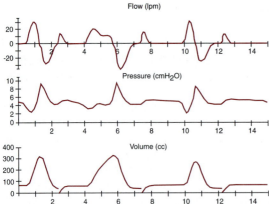

Figure 3-7. CPAP scalars.

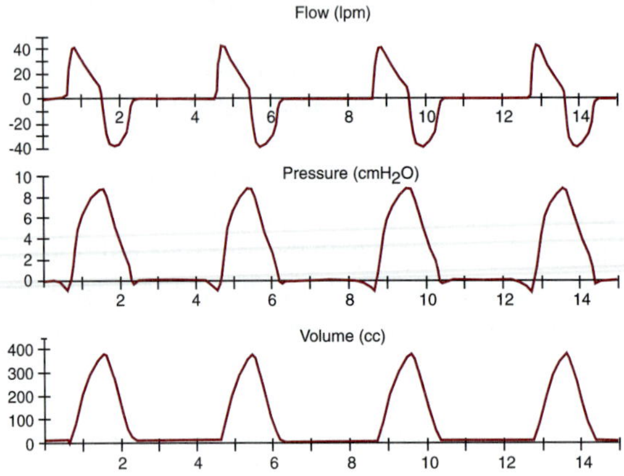

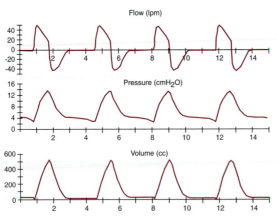

Figure 3-8. PSV scalars.

Figure 3-9. PSV with CPAP scalars.

SPONTANEOUS WAVEFORMS

CONTINUOUS POSITIVE AIRWAY PRESSURE (CPAP): A commonly employed mode used to increase functional residual capacity (FRC) in patients demonstrating refractory hypoxemia. In obstructive sleep apnea, CPAP assists in opening the upper airways.

WAVEFORM CHARACTERISTICS: (Figure 3-7) **Flow/time** curve simply indicates inspiratory and expiratory spontaneous flows**. Pressure/time** is the tracing that identifies the presence of CPAP, which is the spontaneous ventilation baseline maintained at a positive pressure. **Volume/time** shows variable spontaneous volumes.

PRESSURE SUPPORT VENTILATION: This mode augments a spontaneous breath by applying a pre-selected booster pressure to deliver higher volume at a lower patient effort. Most suitable to overcome the work of breathing associated with artificial airways and ventilator circuitry during a spontaneous breath.

WAVEFORM CHARACTERISTICS: (Figure 3-8) **Flow/time** waveform is used to recognize a pressure supported breath. The descending flow waveform abruptly drops to baseline at a system-specific terminal flow (more clearly seen in Figure 3-9). **Pressure/time** tracing indicates a patient triggered breath. The pressure rises to the preset level and plateaus until the flow cycling occurs. **Volume/time** shows delivered volume which depends on the pressure support level.

PSV with CPAP: A mode used to decrease spontaneous work of breathing and support oxygenation. This mode may be used with or without an endotracheal tube. This mode used without an endotracheal tube is termed as **Non-Invasive Positive Pressure Ventilation (NPPV)**. Common applications include home care use in exacerbated COPD patients, sleep apnea patients non responsive to CPAP therapy, and nocturnal ventilatory assistance to restrictive disease patients.

WAVEFORM CHARACTERISTICS: (Figure 3-9) **Flow/time** tracing is similar to flow/time pressure support-only tracing. CPAP is not detected in this scalar. **Pressure/time** scalar identifies an elevated baseline (CPAP) and pressure support level. **Volume/time** waveform is consistent in this example but can vary depending on patient effort.

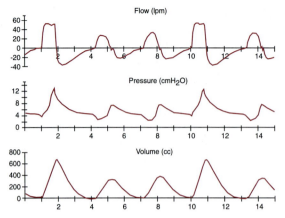

Figure 3-10. Volume-targeted SIMV with CPAP scalars.

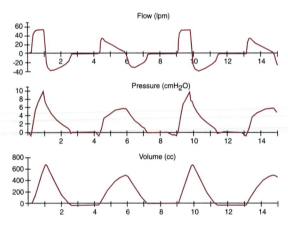

Figure 3-11. Volume-targeted SIMV with PSV scalars.

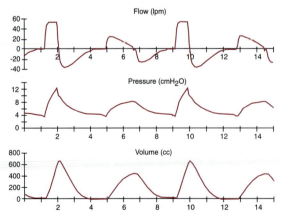

Figure 3-12. Volume-targeted SIMV with CPAP and PSV scalars.

VOLUME-TARGETED VENTILATION

VOLUME-TARGETED SIMV with CPAP: Delivery of SIMV breaths at a higher baseline pressure. Each breath, mechanical or spontaneous, is patient triggered and maintains a clinician selected positive pressure. Patients in hypoxemic respiratory failure, unresponsive to oxygen therapy may benefit from SIMV and CPAP.
WAVEFORM CHARACTERISTICS: (Figure 3-10) **Flow/time** curves indicate the same pattern as SIMV-only. The mechanical and spontaneous breaths are displayed at a higher baseline pressure. **Volume/time** tracing is similar to a SIMV volume waveform.

VOLUME-TARGETED SIMV with PSV: The spontaneous breaths are augmented by an addition of pressure support. All breaths are patient triggered.
WAVEFORM CHARACTERISTICS: (Figure 3-11) **Flow/time** graph demonstrates square flow pattern for mechanical breaths. **The flow/time tracing is the best way to identify pressure-supported breaths.** The pressure supported breaths are indicated by the decreasing flow pattern. The spontaneously triggered (patient triggered) pressure supported breaths are flow cycled whereas the mechanical breaths are volume cycled. **Pressure/time** scalar demonstrates two distinct pressure/time waveforms during a SIMV breath and a pressure supported breath. The PSV breath illustrates a more rounded pressure curve as compared with the smooth rising pressure during the inspiratory phase of the SIMV breath. The presence of PSV is noted on the flow/time scalar whereas the pressure/time scalar indicates PSV and CPAP. **Volume/time** curve indicates the volume differences during the two breaths.

VOLUME-TARGETED SIMV with CPAP and PSV: This mode allows delivery of SIMV and PS breaths at a higher baseline pressure.
WAVEFORM CHARACTERISTICS: (Figure 3-12) **Flow/time** tracing is similar to SIMV with PSV scalar. **Pressure/time** waveform identifies presence of CPAP. **Volume/time** scalar is similar to the SIMV and PSV scalar.

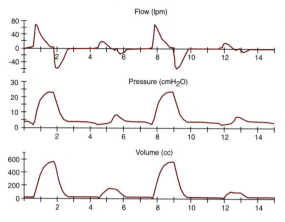

Figure 3-13. Pressure-targeted SIMV with CPAP.

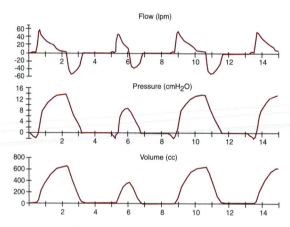

Figure 3-14. Pressure-targeted SIMV with PSV.

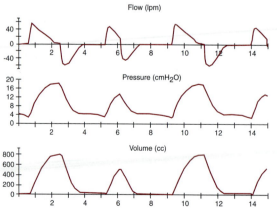

Figure 3-15. Pressure-targeted SIMV with CPAP and PSV.

PRESSURE-TARGETED VENTILATION

PRESSURE-TARGETED SIMV with CPAP: Delivery of SIMV breaths at a higher baseline pressure. Each mechanical breath is an assisted pressure controlled breath (time cycled) interposed by spontaneous breaths. Each breath is patient triggered. The mechanical breaths are delivered at a pre-selected positive pressure.
WAVEFORM CHARACTERISTICS: (Figure 3-13) **Flow/time** scalar indicates the same pattern as SIMV in pressure targeted ventilation. **Pressure/time** tracing indicates CPAP pressure. The pressure tracing does not return to zero. Throughout the cycle, mechanical and spontaneous breaths are displayed at a higher baseline pressure. **Volume/time** scalar is similar to the SIMV only volume scalar.

PRESSURE-TARGETED SIMV with PSV: Spontaneous breaths are augmented by an addition of pre-selected pressure. All breaths are patient triggered.
WAVEFORM CHARACTERISTICS: (Figure 3-14) **Flow/time** graph demonstrates characteristic descending flow pattern for both the pressure control mechanical breaths and pressure support breaths. Observe that in a pressure controlled breath the flow descends steadily until the baseline is reached, followed by a short no-flow state. Whereas in the pressure support breath, the flow descends to a point where inspiration terminates and then flow abruptly drops to the baseline. **The flow/time tracing is the best way to identify pressure controlled and pressure supported breaths.**
Pressure/time scalar demonstrates the two distinct pressure/time waveforms--a pressure targeted SIMV breath and a pressure supported breath. **Volume/time** curve simply indicates the volume differences during the two breaths. In fact if the pressure level is adjusted to match the tidal volume delivered during the SIMV breath (PSV_{max}) the volume/time curve would not show any difference in delivered volumes.

PRESSURE-TARGETED SIMV with CPAP and PSV: This mode allows a delivery of SIMV breaths at a higher baseline pressure and pressure support level.
WAVEFORM CHARACTERISTICS: (Figure 3-15) **Flow/time** tracing is exactly like the SIMV (pressure targeted) with PSV mode and does not give any clue regarding the CPAP addition. **Pressure/time** waveform clearly identifies presence of CPAP and the magnitude of CPAP. The presence of PSV is noted on the flow/time scalar whereas the pressure/time scalar indicates PSV and CPAP. **Volume/time** scalar is identical to the volume/time scalar seen with SIMV with PSV tracing.

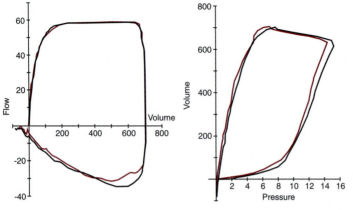

Figure 3-16. Volume-targeted control ventilation loops.

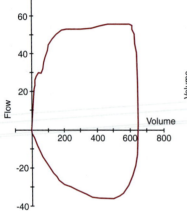
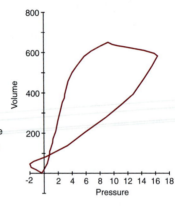

Figure 3-17. Volume-targeted assist/control ventilation loops.

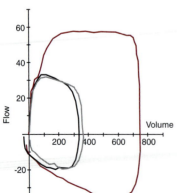
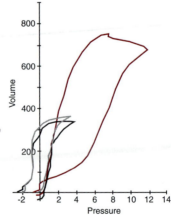

Figure 3-18. Volume-targeted SIMV ventilation loops.

VOLUME-TARGETED VENTILATION
PRESSURE -VOLUME AND FLOW-VOLUME LOOPS

VOLUME-TARGETED CONTROLLED VENTILATION WITH A CONSTANT FLOW: (Figure 3-16) **Flow-Volume loop (F-V)** demonstrates a square wave flow pattern during inspiration (above the volume axis) and exhalation is shown in the bottom part of the loop. The flow quickly increases from zero to the preset peak flow rate and remains unchanged until the inspiratory phase is terminated when the preset tidal volume is delivered (volume- cycled ventilation). Upon termination of inspiration the flow decreases past the baseline to the level of peak expiratory flow rate then ends upon return to the baseline (zero flow). **Pressure-Volume loop (P-V)** represents a loop characterized by constant volume delivery. The tracing begins at the zero origin and concludes at the same point.

VOLUME-TARGETED ASSISTED VENTILATION WITH A CONSTANT FLOW: (Figure 3-17) **F-V loop** is similar to the control mode loop. **P-V loop** illustrates patient triggering. The loop begins at zero. When the loop moves to the left of the volume axis this indicates an inspiratory effort made by the patient. When this effort is detected by the ventilator a mechanical breath is delivered. The loop then moves to the right of the volume axis and returns to zero during exhalation. A spontaneous P-V loop is traced in a clockwise fashion and a mechanical breath is traced counterclockwise. The negative movement to the right of the volume axis represents patient assist (pressure) by the ventilator.

VOLUME-TARGETED SIMV: (Figure 3-18) **F-V loop** shows two levels of loop. The smaller, inner loop represents spontaneous breaths with smaller volumes whereas the larger loop represents a mechanical breath. **P-V loop** tracing includes a smaller P-V loop representing spontaneous breathing (which would be a clockwise tracing on the negative side of the pressure axis). The larger loop illustrates a mechanical breath.

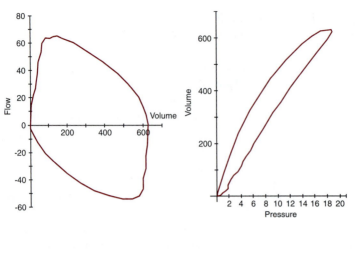

Figure 3-19. Pressure-targeted control ventilation loops.

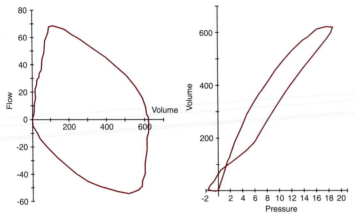

Figure 3-20. Pressure-targeted assist/control ventilation loops.

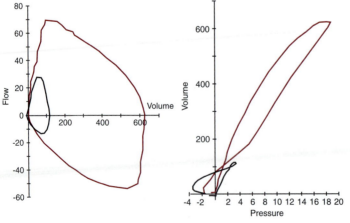

Figure 3-21. Pressure-targeted SIMV loops.

PRESSURE-TARGETED VENTILATION
PRESSURE-VOLUME AND FLOW-VOLUME LOOPS

PRESSURE-TARGETED CONTROLLED VENTILATION: (Figure 3-19) Pressure control mode delivers a time triggered, pressure limited, time cycled ventilation. The inspiratory flow descends during inspiration to maintain the target pressure until the preset inspiratory time elapses. The expiratory flow is descending. **F-V loop** illustrates descending inspiratory as well as expiratory flows. **P-V loop** demonstrates a smaller (thinner) hysteresis as compared to volume ventilation with constant flow. The descending flow is responsible for the smaller hysteresis of the P-V loop.

PRESSURE-TARGETED ASSISTED VENTILATION: (Figure 3-20) Pressure control ventilation in assist mode delivers a patient- triggered, pressure- limited, time-cycled breath. **F-V loop** shows a tracing similar to control ventilation, a descending pattern in both inspiration and expiration. **P-V loop** indicates a negative deflection on the pressure axis consistent with the triggering effort made by the patient.

PRESSURE-TARGETED SIMV: (Figure 3-21) **F-V loop** shows two magnitudes. A smaller loop represents a spontaneous breath and a larger loop illustrating a mechanical breath. **P-V loop** also illustrates a smaller spontaneous loop and a larger loop associated with a mechanical breath. The small negative pressure loop represents the patient's effort to trigger the machine breath. The slightly larger loop encompassing the smaller negative pressure loop represents the spontaneous breath. The largest loop on the positive pressure side represents the machine breath.

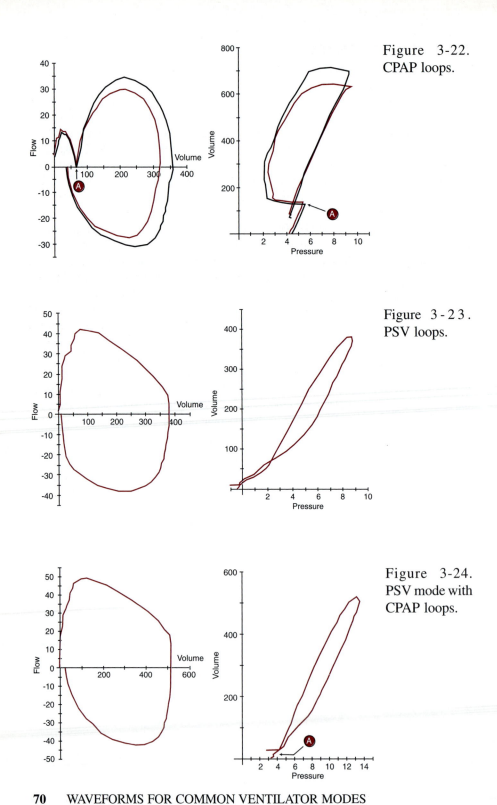

Figure 3-22. CPAP loops.

Figure 3-23. PSV loops.

Figure 3-24. PSV mode with CPAP loops.

SPONTANEOUS BREATHS
P-V AND F-V LOOPS

CPAP: (Figure 3-22) **F-V loop** shows some deviation from the zero volume point during exhalation due to a leak in the circuit. At the beginning of inspiration the flow rate drops momentarily to zero (item A) before completing inspiration. CPAP is not reflected on the F-V loop. **P-V loop** clearly illustrates that the pressure volume tracing originates at a higher pressure and returns to nearly the same point at the end of the breath. This pressure variance is indicative of CPAP. Item A in the P-V loop corresponds to item A in the F-V loop. Volume increases briefly with a positive increase in pressure and then pressure decreases for the remainder of inspiration. This type of inspiratory beginning is likely due to an aggressive flow compensation setting.

PSV: (Figure 3-23) **F-V loop** illustrates a descending inspiratory flow rate until a system-specific flow is achieved, then the flow rate rapidly decreases to zero. The expiratory portion of the loop continues until the lung volume and flow return to zero. **P-V loop** illustrates patient-triggering, then the pressure support breath is delivered with expiration returning to zero baseline. The loop moves in a clockwise pattern during the initial phase (patient-triggering) of the pressure support breath and then counterclockwise for the mechanically delivered pressurized breath.

PSV with CPAP: (Figure 3-24) **F-V loop** tracing representing PSV and CPAP shows congruence to figure 3-23 which represents the F-V loop for PSV mode. **P-V loop** is similar to P-V loop for PSV except the point of origin and the point of termination for this loop is at a higher pressure level indicating CPAP.

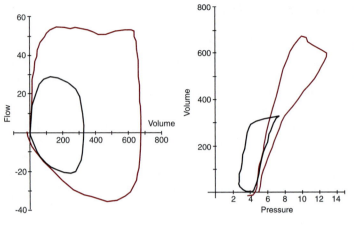

Figure 3-25. Volume-targeted SIMV with CPAP loops.

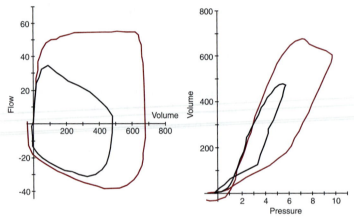

Figure 3-26. Volume-targeted SIMV with PS loops.

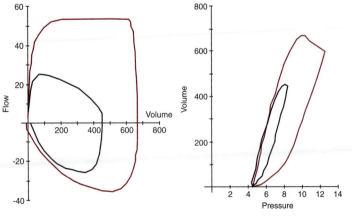

Figure 3-27. Volume-targeted SIMV with PS loops and CPAP.

VOLUME-TARGETED VENTILATION

VOLUME-TARGETED SIMV with CPAP: (Figure 3-25) **F-V loop** is similar to Figure 3-18 indicating two distinct loops, one a mechanical breath and the other a spontaneous breath. **P-V loop** has a similar appearance as Figure 3-18, except that the zero point is moved to a positive pressure level consistent with CPAP.

VOLUME-TARGETED SIMV with PSV: (Figure 3-26) **F-V loop** shows two types of tracings; a PSV tracing (smaller loop) and a mechanical breath (larger loop). The mechanical breath is an assisted breath similar to Figure 3-17. **P-V loop** is essentially a combination of a tracing similar to Figure 3-23 superimposed onto Figure 3-17. The two breaths are separate types and seeing them together in Figure 3-26 provides practice in distinguishing the two.

VOLUME-TARGETED SIMV with PSV and CPAP: (Figure 3-27) **F-V loop** does not indicate any presence of CPAP. It shows a similar pattern as the F-V loop in Figure 3-26. **P-V loop** is similar to Figure 3-26 except CPAP is present.

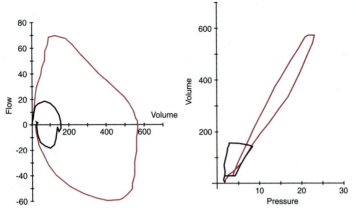

Figure 3-28. Pressure-targeted SIMV with CPAP loops.

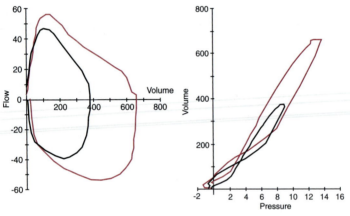

Figure 3-29. Pressure-targeted SIMV with PS loops.

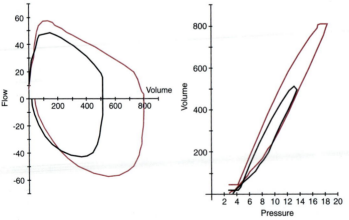

Figure 3-30. Pressure-targeted SIMV with PS loops and CPAP.

PRESSURE-TARGETED VENTILATION

PRESSURE-TARGETED SIMV with CPAP: (Figure 3-28) The SIMV breath begins at a higher baseline pressure indicating the presence of CPAP. **F-V loop:** Distinct loops representing an SIMV breath in pressure control mode similar to Figure 3-21 and a spontaneous breath. **P-V loop** has a similar appearance to the P-V loop in Figure 3-21, except for the higher baseline pressure representing CPAP.

PRESSURE-TARGETED SIMV with PSV: (Figure 3-29) This figure shows two types of tracings; a PSV tracing and a mechanical breath. The mechanical breath (higher volume and flow tracing) is an assisted breath similar to Figure 3-20. The smaller loop represents a PS breath similar to Figure 3-23. **P-V loop** provides a tracing that would be similar to superimposing Figure 3-20 onto Figure 3-23. The larger loop represents the machine breath and the smaller loop represents the PS breath.

PRESSURE-TARGETED SIMV with PSV and CPAP: (Figure 3-30) **F-V loop** does not indicate any presence of CPAP. It shows an identical pattern as the F-V loop in Figure 3-29. **P-V loop** is similar to Figure 3-29 except the zero point is advanced to a higher level illustrating a presence of CPAP.

CHAPTER 4
COMMON CLINICAL FINDINGS

I.   Changes in Respiratory System Compliance
                Decreased Compliance
                Inflection Points
                Overdistension
                Active Exhalation

II.   Airway Obstruction
                Bronchospasm: Bronchodilator Benefit Assessment
                Air-Trapping
                        Dynamic Hyperinflation
                        Early Small Airway Collapse
                Kinked Endotracheal Tube

III.   Patient-Ventilator Dys-synchrony
                Inadequate Inspiratory Flow Rate
                Inappropriate Trigger Sensitivity
                Patient and Ventilator Rates Out of Synchrony

IV.   Leaks

There are many possible abnormal ventilator waveform variations but the most common findings make a relatively short list. The following specific examples are arranged under the general categories to which they relate.

CHANGES IN RESPIRATORY SYSTEM COMPLIANCE
DECREASED COMPLIANCE

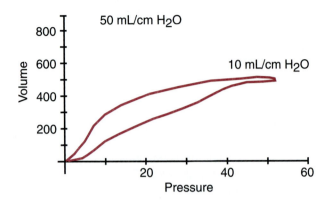

Figure 4-1. The P-V loop of a patient with severely decreased respiratory compliance.

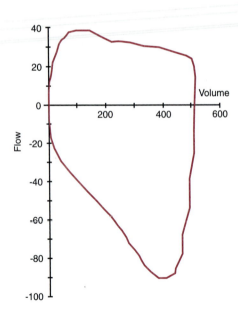

Figure 4-2. The F-V loop of a patient with severely decreased respiratory compliance.

Decreased respiratory compliance is best appreciated in the P-V loop (Figure 4-1). The black line indicates the slope of the value for the low-end of the normal compliance range. The loop has a dynamic compliance of 10 mL/cm H_2O and is shifted downward and to the right of the normal compliance line. The F-V loop corresponding to this patient example is essentially normal except for the relatively high expiratory flow rate for a tidal volume of 500 mL (Figure 4-2). The F-V loop does not provide much information for this particular patient condition but it is given in this instance for orientation purposes.

Patients with conditions that lead to alveolar instability such as acute respiratory distress syndrome often have increased alveolar collapse during exhalation and a decreased FRC. The collapsed alveoli must be reinflated at the beginning of the next breath at a significant cost in

INFLECTION POINTS

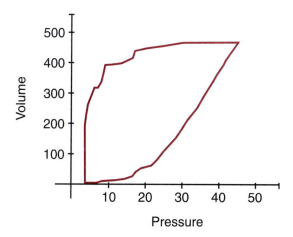

Figure 4-3. An example of an abnormal inflection point at the beginning of inspiration in a P-V loop due to alveolar instability.

terms of increased ventilating pressure (Figure 4-3). This produces increased shear forces that eventually cause further lung injury. PEEP is applied to maintain the patency of compromised alveoli. Figure 4-4 shows the results of raising the PEEP from 5 to 12 cm H_2O. The tidal volume remains essentially the same with little change in the PIP. The pressure change (PIP-PEEP) is actually less with 12 cm H_2O of PEEP and the dynamic compliance (PIP-PEEP/tidal volume) is improved.

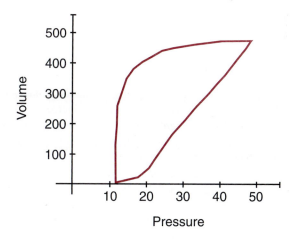

Figure 4-4. The effect of PEEP on a P-V loop with an abnormal inspiratory inflection point due to alveolar instability.

OVERDISTENSION

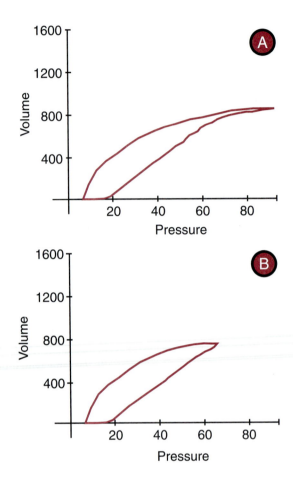

Figure 4-5. Identification and correction of overdistension as seen in P-V loops.

Overdistension occurs when the volume capacity of the lungs has been exceeded and the application of additional pressure causes very little increase in volume (loop A in Figure 4-5). The volume limit is identified on the P-V loop as an abrupt change in compliance in the terminal portion of inspiration, a second inspiratory inflection point. This abnormal loop shape is commonly termed "beaking" and results in a reduced slope having a decreased dynamic compliance. Overdistension can lead to volutrauma, particularly in lung regions with normal alveoli. Correction of overdistension involves decreasing the pressure setting in pressure-targeted ventilation or decreasing the volume setting in volume-targeted ventilation. The loop in graph B shows that a small decrease in the set tidal volume produced a large decrease in the PIP.

ACTIVE EXHALATION

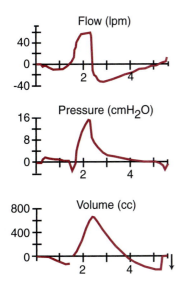

Figure 4-6. Active exhalation displayed in scalars.

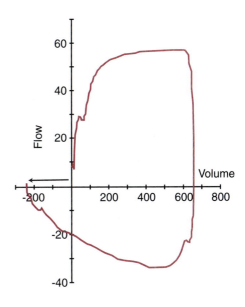

Figure 4-7. Active exhalation displayed in F-V loop.

When a patient exhales more than the inspiratory volume, active exhalation has occurred. The waveforms in Figures 4-6, 4-7, and 4-8 show active exhalation of an additional volume of about 200 ml. For expiratory volume to be greater than inspiratory volume, the patient has to exhale below FRC. It is normal for this to happen occasionally in the clinical setting for example, when the patient changes position, experiences a twinge of pain, or tries to resist an urge to cough. It is not normal if it happens in a regular pattern. Patients with air-trapping will often show a pattern of an active exhalation occurring every few breaths in attempt to relieve the trapped volume. A larger expiratory volume than inspiratory volume on every breath indicates the expiratory flow transducer is out of calibration or some other equipment error exists.

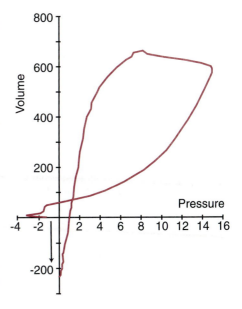

Figure 4-8. Active exhalation displayed in P-V loop.

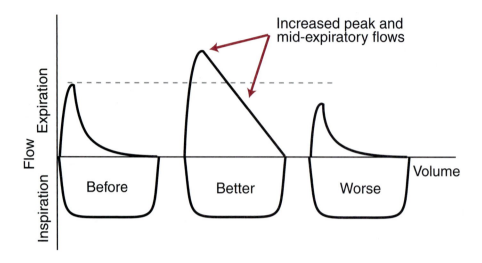

Figure 4-9. Indicators of airway improvement in the F-V loop as a result of response to a bronchodilator.

The effects of a bronchodilator are best appreciated in the F-V loop (Figure 4-9). The two major changes that indicate improvement are an increased peak expiratory flow rate and an increased mid-expiratory flow rate. Decreased mid-expiratory flow rates produce a "scooped" appearance in the descending portion of the expiratory curve ("Before" and "Worse" loops in Figure 4-9). An improvement from bronchodilator will yield an increased tidal volume in pressure-targeted ventilation and sometimes in volume-targeted ventilation. An example of a positive bronchodilator response is given in Figure 4-10. Loop B shows increased peak and mid-expiratory flow rates compared to the pretreatment loop A.

Response to bronchodilator can also be seen in P-V loops. Loop B in Figure 4-11 shows decreased loop hysteresis compared to loop A. The maximal volume is slightly increased in this volume-targeted breath. Pressure-targeted ventilation tends to show similar and often more pronounced pre- and post-bronchodilator changes in the P-V loop given the same lung conditions. It is very useful to store a pre- and post-bronchodilator F-V loop in computer memory or print them for comparison. Comparing pre- and post-bronchodilator loops in one's memory is unreliable. It is best to keep the same axis scaling for both measurements if possible for ease of comparison.

Lack of response to bronchodilator may indicate that increased airways resistance is not due to bronchospasm. Airway narrowing may be due to fluid in the airways or swelling of the mucosa due to an inflammatory process not responsive to beta$_2$ agonists or parasympatholytic agents. Pre- and post-loops after a trial of steroids may be help-

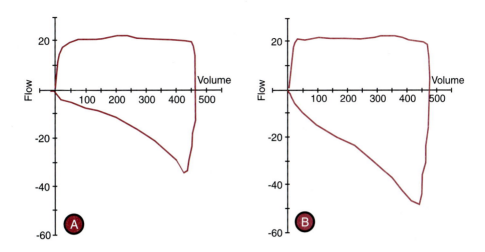

Figure 4-10. Pre- and post-bronchodilator F-V loops of volume-targeted breaths.

ful for guiding therapy. Pre- and post loops can also be used for assessing which type of bronchodilator works best for a particular patient or if some combination of drugs has a superior effect. A post-drug loop that is worse than the pre-drug loop may indicate the patient is reacting to the drug propellent or preservative.

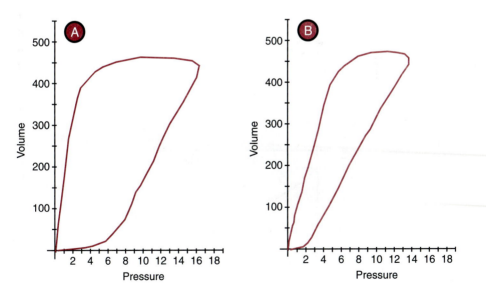

Figure 4-11. Pre- and post-bronchodilator P-V loops of volume-targeted breaths.

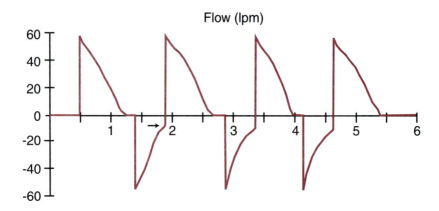

Figure 4-12. Flow scalar showing air-trapping due to dynamic hyperinflation.

Air-trapping and the associated auto-PEEP is generally caused by two mechanisms, dynamic hyperinflation and early collapse of unstable airways during exhalation. Dynamic hyperinflation occurs when the respiratory rate does not allow sufficient time for complete exhalation before the next breath. Figure 4-12 demonstrates this condition with early termination of exhalation indicated by the arrow. A similar example of early termination of exhalation is shown in the F-V loop of Figure 4-13. If dynamic hyperinflation is due to an excessive patient-triggered respiratory rate it may be helpful

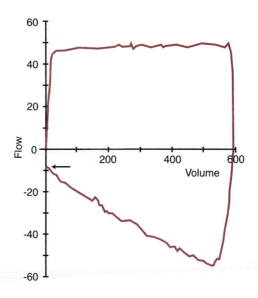

Figure 4-13. Air-trapping identified in the F-V loop of a volume-targeted breath.

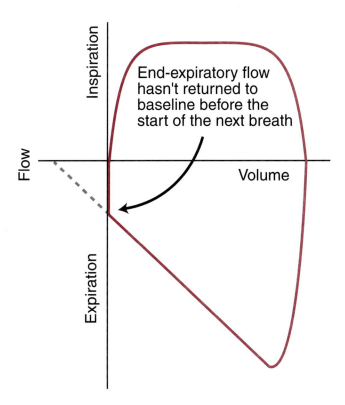

Figure 4-14. Conceptual illustration of why the F-V loop is altered by air-trapping.

to switch to SIMV mode or if necessary, sedate the patient. If a high respiratory rate is necessary and dynamic hyperinflation occurs, especially when bronchospasm is also present, increasing the inspiratory peak flow rate may yield improvement by extending the time for exhalation.

To better understand why the F-V loop changes shape at the end of exhalation a conceptualized rendering is given in Figure 4-14. If expiratory time was extended the loop would follow the path of the gray dashed line. Instead, the loop returns abruptly to the baseline at the start of the next breath. The potential additional volume is exaggerated in this example to clarify the concept of air-trapping. In reality the loop would not necessarily trace a straight line if expiratory time was extended but additional volume would be measured. It is important to note that these examples only detect the presence of air-trapping and do not quantify it in cm H_2O.

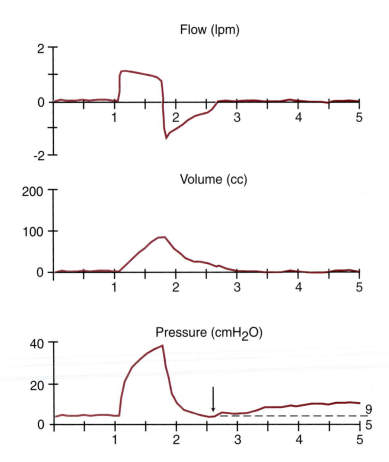

Figure 4-15. Measurement of auto-PEEP in a patient with early airways collapse during expiration.

The other cause of air-trapping relates to the early collapse of small airways during expiration. Lung diseases that cause destruction of normal airway structure result in tissue being replaced by scar tissue that collapses more easily. This results in early airway closure during expiration. Auto-PEEP associated with air-trapping can be measured by using either of two clinical techniques. The dynamic technique requires the simultaneous measurement of esophageal pressure and will not be addressed here. The second technique involves measuring the airway pressure while occluding the expiratory side of the ventilator circuit near end exhalation (Figure 4-15). The end-expiratory occlusion technique for measuring auto-PEEP requires sufficient expiratory time for the occlusion pressure to reach a plateau or the value will not be accurate. Patient respiratory efforts during the expiratory occlusion will also interfere with accurate measurements.

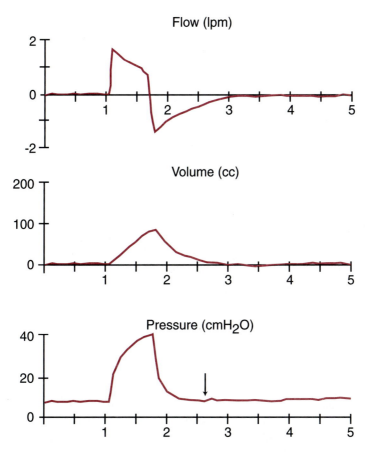

Figure 4-16. Application of external PEEP to correct auto-PEEP caused by early airways collapse during expiration.

The end-expiratory occlusion technique is displayed in Figure 4-15. The arrow indicates the occlusion of the expiratory circuit after the tracing has reached baseline (PEEP of 5 cm H_2O). The airway pressure tracing rises and eventually plateaus at a level of 14 cm H_2O. This represents 5 cm H_2O of PEEP and 9 cm H_2O of auto-PEEP. Correction of this auto-PEEP is attempted in Figure 4-16. The external PEEP was increased to 8 cm H_2O and the end-expiratory occlusion measurement now indicates an acceptable 2 cm H_2O of auto-PEEP.

KINKED ENDOTRACHEAL TUBE

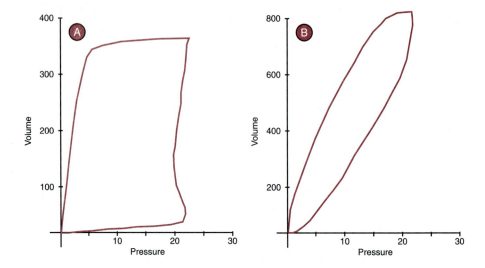

Figure 4-17. The effect of a kinked endotracheal tube on the P-V loop during pressure-targeted ventilation.

A kinked endotracheal tube (ETT) can occur suddenly or gradually. When passing a suction catheter through the ETT becomes difficult, the possibility of a partially obstructed ETT should be considered. This condition is a type of upper airway obstruction, shown in loop A of Figure 4-17. Note the considerable hysteresis and low tidal volume associated with a PIP of 22 cm H_2O. Attempts to reposition the ETT and the patient's head were unsuccessful at relieving the obstruction because a memory of bend in the tubing had developed. Loop B shows the resolution of the obstruction after replacement of the ETT. Partial obstruction of an artificial airway can also be caused by dried secretions or blood in the lumen or at the end of the tube.

PATIENT-VENTILATOR DYS-SYNCHRONY
INADEQUATE INSPIRATORY FLOW RATE

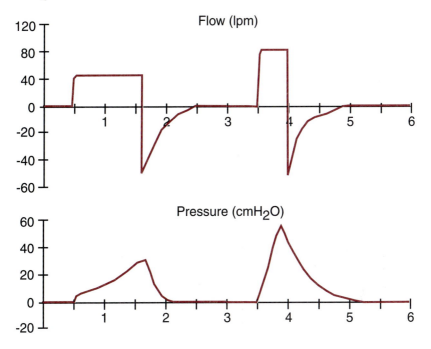

Figure 4-18. Dys-synchrony due to flow starvation.

Setting the peak inspiratory flow rate optimally in volume-targeted ventilation is often overlooked. This simple adjustment can improve patient comfort in general and especially when resting a patient on the ventilator who is being weaned by increasing periods of spontaneous breathing. The pressure scalar of the first breath in Figure 4-18 shows flow starvation, a concave or downward-scooped curve during inspiratory phase. The peak flow rate was increased in the second breath to better match the patient's inspiratory demand. Increasing the peak flow worked in this example it but setting the flow too high can produce turbulence that may lead to pressure-limiting.

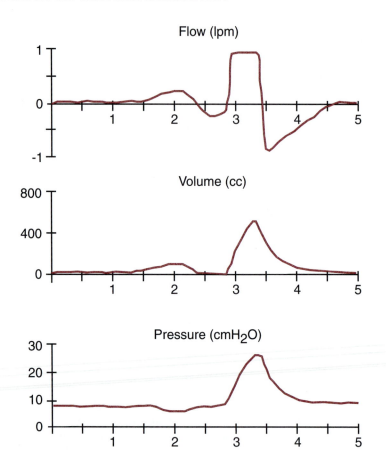

Figure 4-19. Failure to trigger a machine breath in response to patient inspiratory efforts due to an inappropriate sensitivity setting.

The three scalars in Figure 4-19 all show signs of patient effort around the two second time mark but no machine breath was triggered. Although the pressure drop due to the patient's effort was not large, it was sustained for nearly a second. The patient's diaphragmatic strength may be marginal. Continued unsatisfied patient efforts can lead to patient anxiety further compromise of the diaphragm.

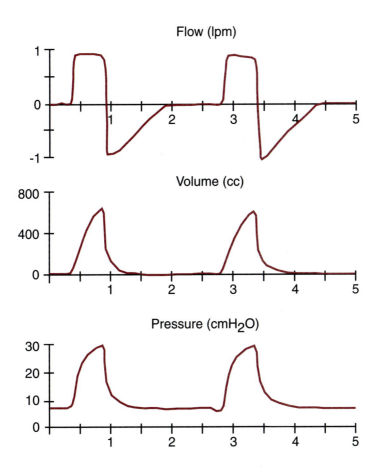

Figure 4-20. Ventilator sensitivity increased to allow for ventilator response to patient inspiratory efforts.

The first breath in Figure 4-20 was untriggered, indicated by the lack of pressure or flow change immediately prior to the machine breath. The second breath is an assisted breath as indicated by the slight pressure deflection before the machine breath. The sensitivity has been increased so that a machine breath is triggered before the patient can generate the magnitude of spontaneous effort observed in Figure 4-19.

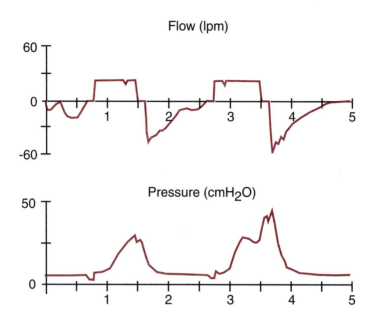

Figure 4-21. Patient rate and ventilator rate out of synchrony.

Patient/ventilator rate dys-synchony can have several causes. A patient may have a very high spontaneous rate due to a sensation of air hunger or as a result of a neurologic injury. Aside from the acid-base and air-trapping problems that can occur from supporting a high respiratory rate, if compliance and resistance are normal the machine breaths may remain synchronous with the patient up to a point. Beyond that point patient and machine patterns become uncoupled. Patients with neurologic injury can become uncoupled from the ventilator pattern even at normal spontaneous rates.

Clinicians sometimes confuse rate dys-snychrony with flow-starvation (Figure 4-18). Unlike flow starvation the scalars in Figure 4-21 show abnormal patterns in the expiratory phase as well as the inspiratory phase. Also, the abnormal pattern changes from breath to breath whereas the pattern for flow starvation is typically similar for each breath.

Choosing a ventilatory mode/s with rapid initial delivery such as PCV with PSV can often help minimize this type dys-synchrony. Fine-tuning the ventilator to the patient in this fashion will hopefully decrease the need for patient sedation. Some patients requiring full ventilatory support are difficult to synchronize with even using PCV and may respond best to just PSV. The pressure level can be titrated to best match the patient's pattern within the range needed for adequate gas exchange. Apnea ventilation parameters must be properly set before attempting such a trial.

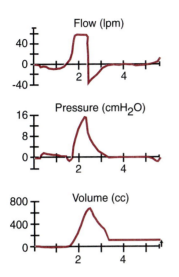

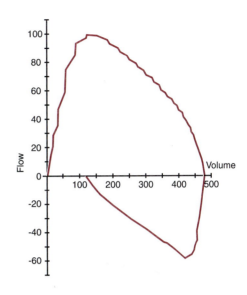

Figure 4-22. Volume loss displayed in a volume scalar.

Figure 4-23. Volume loss displayed in a F-V loop.

Volume leaks can be easily detected in the volume scalar, F-V loop, and P-V loop. The volume scalar of Figure 4-22 does not return to the baseline during exhalation for the displayed breath. A plateau above the zero volume baseline is created by the lost volume (arrow). Volume loss is detected in the F-V and P-V loops as a failure to close the loops (Figures 4-23 and 4-24). Inspiratory and expiratory volume should be the same but will vary slightly even under normal conditions due to momentary changes in patient lung conditions, cuff seal, etc. Consistent volume loss should be systematically investigated for correction. A source of leak that is sometimes hard to identify is a misplaced nasogastric tube in the trachea, especially if one is unaware the tube has been replaced. In this situation, expiratory volume loss is accompanied by the patient exerting greater effort to trigger a ventilator breath.

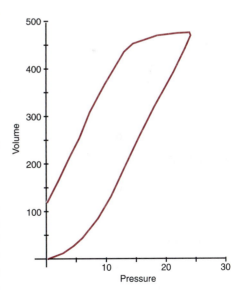

Figure 4-23. Volume loss displayed in a P-V loop.

CHAPTER 5
NEONATAL APPLICATIONS

INTRODUCTION

Mechanical ventilation of neonates and small infants is commonly applied by a time-triggered, pressure-limited, time cycled ventilator. These ventilators have a continuous flow that delivers a specific F_IO_2. During spontaneous breathing the continuous flow provides a fresh gas source to the patient. Mandatory or controlled breaths are based on setting of the inspiratory time (time-cycled) and frequency (time-triggered). When the ventilator time-triggers a breath a signal is sent to the exhalation valve to close. Flow (decelerating flow curve) enters the patient's lungs through the inspiratory limb of the patient circuit for the set inspiratory time. When pressure reaches the set limit the remaining pressure is diverted to a limited device. As the ventilator cycles the exhalation valve opens and allows the patient volume and continuous flow to exit. Tidal volume delivered by the ventilator depends on the pressure limit, inspiratory time, flow rate, and positive end-expiratory pressure (PEEP). The amount of volume entering the lungs depends on lung and chest-wall compliance, resistance of the endotracheal tube, and airways.

Over the past few years neonatal ventilation has become more sophisticated incorporating into the ventilators new modes of ventilation such as synchronize intermittent mandatory ventilation (SIMV) and synchronized assist control ventilation and bedside respiratory mechanical monitoring. Respiratory monitoring gives the practitioner at the bedside the ability to monitor infants more effectively, identify abnormalities between the patient and ventilator and intervene to provide optimal ventilatory care. In spite of these improvements identification of ventilator problems by ventilator graphics is still challenging.

The benefits of bedside respiratory monitoring include recognition of:
1. Asynchronous breathing
2. Breath stacking, air trapping and auto-PEEP
3. Expiratory grunting, prolong expiratory time
4. Change in dynamic compliance from lung disease or administration of surfactant
5. Inadvertent extubation
6. Excessive inspiratory pressure
7. Inappropriate inspiratory flow rate
8. Inappropriate sensitivity setting
9. Excessive inspiratory time
10. Excessive inspiratory flow rate
11. Excessive endotracheal tube leak

NORMAL INFANT PULMONARY FUNCTIONS

Measurement Term	Units	Normal	RDS	BPD
Tidal volume	mL/kg	5-7	4-6	4-7
Respiratory rate	breaths/min	30-60	50-80	45-80
Minute ventilation	mL/kg/min	200-300	250-400	200-400
Function residual capacity (FRC)	mL/kg	20-30	15-20	20-30
Compliance (static)	mL/cm H_2O/kg	1-4	0.1-0.6	0.2-0.8
Compliance (dynamic)	mL/cm H_2O/kg	1-2	0.3-0.5	0.2-0.8
Resistance	cm H_2O/mL/sec	0.025-0.05	0.06-.15	0.03-0.15
Resistance	cm H_2O/L/sec	25-50	60-150	30-150
Work of Breathing	gram/cm/min/kg	500-1000	800-3000	1800-6500
VD/VT ratio	Percent	22-38	60-80	35-60
Dead space	mL/kg	1.0-2.0	3.0-4.5	3.0-4.5
Pulmonary capillary blood flow	mL/kg/min	160-230	75-140	120-200
Oxygen consumption	mL/kg/min	6-8		
CO_2 production	mL/kg/min	5-6		
Respiratory quotient		0.75-0.83		
Calories	kcal/kg/day	105-183		

(Adapted from SensorMedics Corporation, Yorba Linda, California)

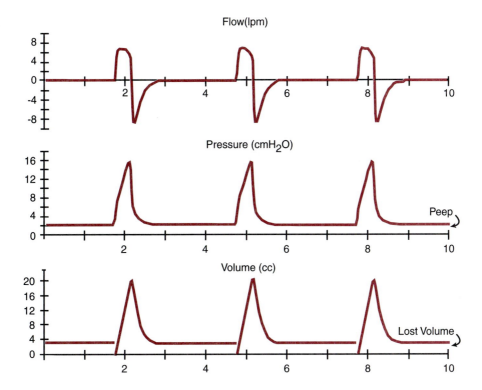

Figure 5-1. Neonatal control ventilation scalars.

The scalars in Figure 5-1 show mandatory or "controlled" breaths delivered by a time-triggered, pressure-limited, time cycled ventilator. The pressure scalar following a positive pressure breath (PPB) returns to baseline pressure of 2 cm H_2O representing PEEP. The driving pressure is 14 cm H_2O (16 cm H_2O - 2 cm H_2O = 14 cm H_2O). These breaths being mandatory breaths show no drop in pressure below baseline that would indicate a spontaneous inspiratory effort by the patient.

The flow scalar shows a flow rate of 8 L/m with a decelerating flow. The exhalation portion of the flow curve returns to baseline before the next breath is delivered. The volume scalar returns to baseline of 3 mL indicating lost volume. This is normal for a patient with a cuff-less endotracheal tube where some volume leaks around the tube as a PPB is delivered to the lungs. Lost volume should not exceed 20% of the total volume delivered. Lost volume here represents 15%.

The F-V loop in Figure 5-2 shows a flow rate of 8 L/m and a delivered volume of 20 mL. The loop rises as flow rate enters the lung and a pressure is reached. That pressure is maintained for the set inspiratory time. When inspiratory time is complete exhalation resulting in loop to move downward. This corresponds to the flow scalar on the exhalation side. The loop returns to baseline. The return volume (exhalation portion of the loop) returns to 3 mL. This represents the lost volume that corresponds to the volume scalar.

The P-V loop in Figure 5-3 shows a pressure of 16 cm H_2O (driving pressure is 14 cm H_2O) delivery and an exhaled volume of 17 mL. The P-V loop starts at 3 cm H_2O representing the level of PEEP set on the ventilator.

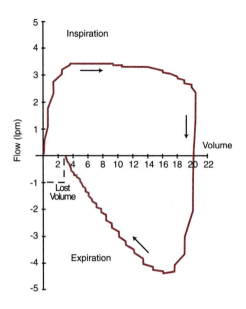

Figure 5-2. Control ventilation flow-volume loop.

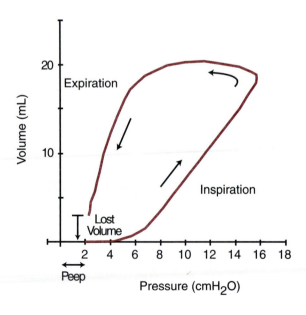

Figure 5-3. Control ventilation pressure-volume loop.

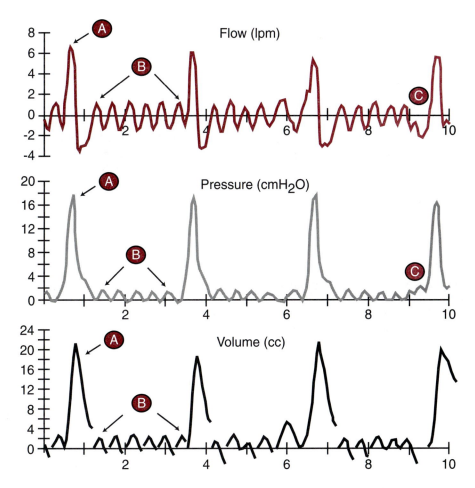

Figure 5-4. IMV scalars.

A patient is receiving pressure-limited, time-cycled, continuous flow ventilation in IMV mode (Figure 5-4). A represents a positive pressure breathing and B represents spontaneous breaths on the flow, pressure, and volume scalar. The first 3 positive pressure breaths are delivered in synchronous with the patient's inspiratory effort. At point C the patient begins to exhale but before complete exhalation occurs a positive pressure breath is delivered . Compare this with SIMV scalars in Figure 5-7.

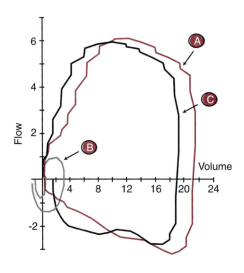

Figure 5-5 shows F-V loops for the segment of breathing shown in Figure 5-4. The mandatory machine breaths are shown in red and black and spontaneous breaths are represented in gray. Because the ventilator in this example used a simple interruption of constant flow to generate breaths, the machine breaths were susceptible to slight alterations by the patient's respiratory efforts.

The P-V loops for respirations in Figure 5-4 are given in Figure 5-6. Note the change in volumes as patient compliance changes from breath to breath.

Figure 5-5. IMV flow-volume loops.

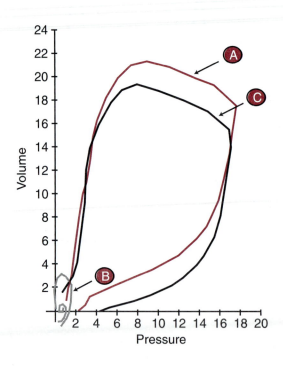

Figure 5-6. IMV pressure-volume loops.

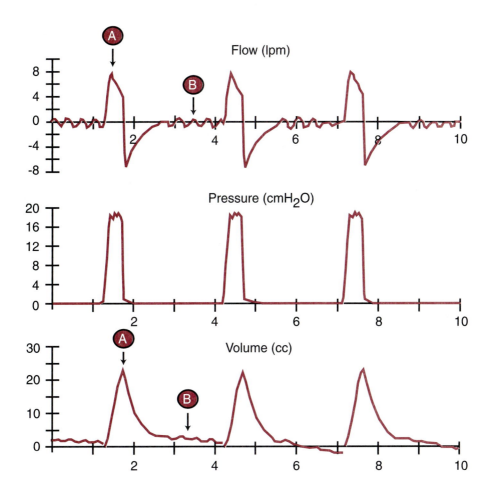

Figure 5-7. Pressure control SIMV scalars.

The patient in Figure 5-7 was receiving pressure-targeted ventilation in the SIMV mode. Point A represents a positive pressure breath. Point B represents spontaneous breaths. Note that end of each series of spontaneous breaths the next positive pressure breath is delivered at end exhalation as seen on the flow scalar as the exhalation portion of the flow curve returns (resets) to baseline.

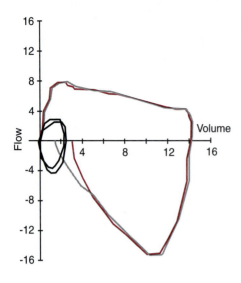

The F-V loops in Figure 5-8 were created with a ventilator in a pressure-targeted mode synchronized with the patient's inspiratory efforts which yielded more uniform machine breaths. Although the volume was fairly constant in example, it can vary according to amount of patient effort in a pressure-targeted mode.

The machine P-V loops in Figure 5-9 clearly indicate a pressure-targeted mode is being used. Inspiratory pressure quickly increases to the set limit and is maintained until the end of the inspiratory period.

Figure 5-8. Pressure control SIMV flow-volume loops.

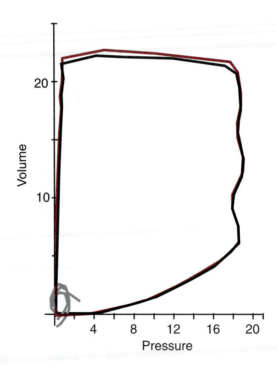

Figure 5-9. Pressure control SIMV pressure-volume loops.

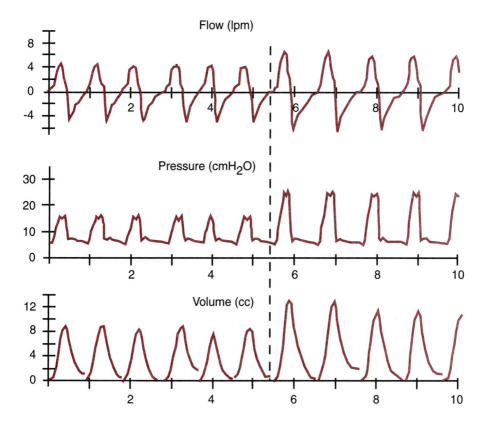

Figure 5-10. Pressure support ventilation of 10 to 20 cm H_2O with CPAP of 5 cm H_2O scalars.

The scalars in Figure 5-10 represent a change in PSV from 10 to 20 cm H_2O with a baseline CPAP of 5 cm H_2O. A PSV level of 10 cm H_2O with a baseline of 5 cm H_2O yields a total pressure of 15 cm H_2O with a driving pressure of 10 cm H_2O (15 cm H_2O - 5 cm H_2O = 10 cm H_2O). When PSV level is increased to 20 cm H_2O, flow and volume increase due to the increase in driving pressure to 20 cm H_2O (25 cm H_2O - 5 cm H_2O = 20 cm H_2O).

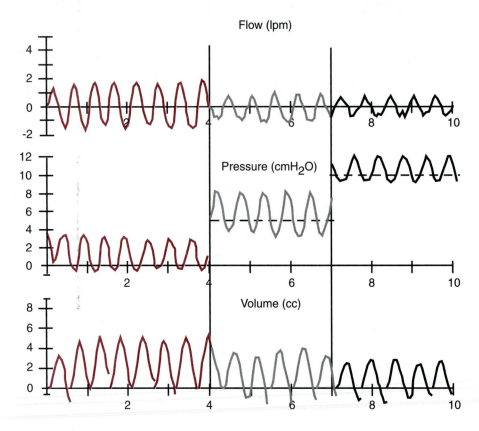

Figure 5-11. Spontaneous ventilation with CPAP scalars.

Scalars in Figure 5-11 show CPAP levels of 0, 5 and 10 cm H_2O. Note how as CPAP is increased to 10 cm H_2O there is a reduction in flow and volume return.

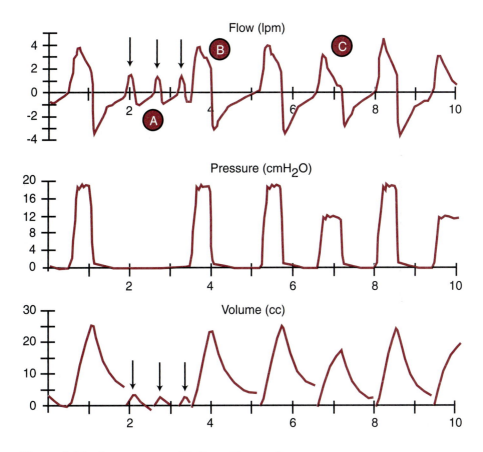

Figure 5-12. Improper sensitivity setting scalars.

The patient in Figure 5-12 is in SIMV mode with PSV. The flow and volume scalars indicated spontaneous breaths at point A. Each arrow represents a spontaneous breath. Note on the pressure scalar there is no pressure deflection. No pressure support breath delivered as the sensitivity on the ventilator is improper for the inspiratory effort of the infant. Point B represents delivery of a positive pressure breath after which the sensitivity was increased. Point C represents a PS breath being delivered as a result of the new sensitivity setting.

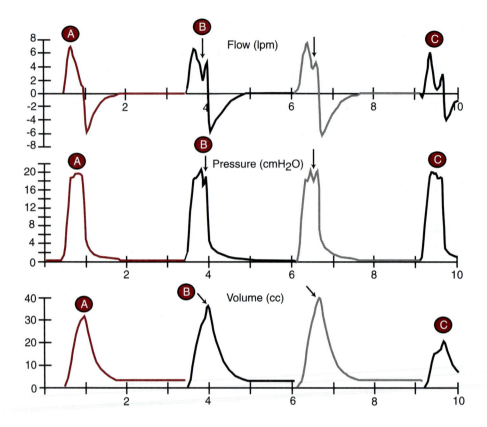

Figure 5-12. A/C pressure control asychrony scalars.

The first breath A on the flow, pressure, and volume scalars represents normal synchronous breathing (Figure 5-12). Compare these waveforms to the next 3 waveforms on
each scalar. On the flow scalar arrows pointing to the notched area during inspiratory
phase indicates an inspiratory effort. Fluctuation in pressure occurs during the inspiratory effort as seen on the pressure scalar. This coincides with fluctuation in flow as the
infant inspires. The volume scalar demonstrates fluctuation in volume. The second
and third volume waveforms show increases in volume as a result of the inspiration
taken during the positive pressure breath. The third volume waveform shows a reduction due to asynchrony.

The loops and numbers in Figures 5-13 and 5-14 correspond with those in Figure 5-12. Inspiratory flow normally follows a decreasing pattern after reaching a peak flow (red loop). Figure 5-13 shows flow increasing and decreasing twice during the inspiratory phase due to patient-ventilator asynchrony (black and gray loops). Asynchrony is seen where flow is decreasing and then an upswing in the flow-volume curve occurs. This is due to the patient initiating another inspiratory effort near the end of the ventilator's inspiratory period. Note the alteration in volume with each breath.

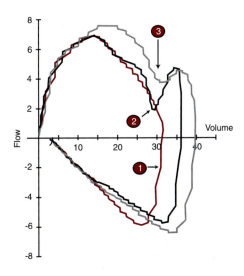

Figure 5-13. AC pressure control asynchrony flow-volume loops.

The P-V loops in Figure 5-14 show a rapid initial rise in pressure as volume enters the lung. Change in the loop occurs as the infant inspires during the inspiratory phase of the positive pressure breath. Each P-V loop can be compared to the scalars in Figure 5-12. Note the change in volume of each P-V loop from 1 to 2, and 2 to 3. The continual rise in pressure to the set point indicates flow is adequate for the patient (red loop).

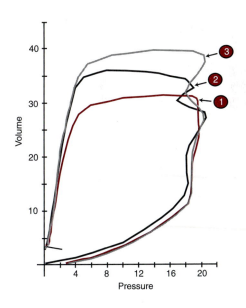

Figure 5-14. AC pressure control asynchrony pressure-volume loops.

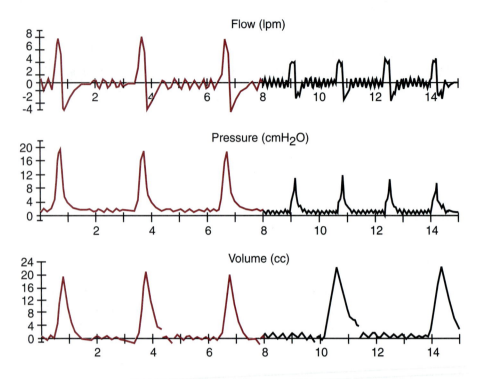

Figure 5-15. Low flow setting scalars.

Inadequate flow produces nonuniform scalar shapes as seen in the flow and pressure scalars of Figure 5-15. The ventilator flow rate is insufficient to achieve the set pressure. This is likely due to insufficient inspiratory time at the lower flow rate setting (a reduction from 7 to 5 L/min from red to black portion of the tracing).

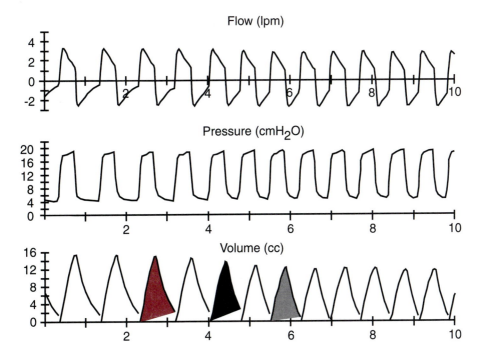

Figure 5-16. Breath-stacking scalars.

A high mechanical ventilator rate can cause breath-stacking to occur. In Figure 5-16, note on the flow scalar how the expiratory flow rate does not reach baseline before the next mechanical breath is delivered. As the mechanical rate is changed (moving from left to right) note how the next positive pressure breath starts earlier. On the volume scalar note how an increase in respiratory rate causes volume to decrease. Each new breath is stacked on top of the preceding breath causing air to remain trapped in the lung.

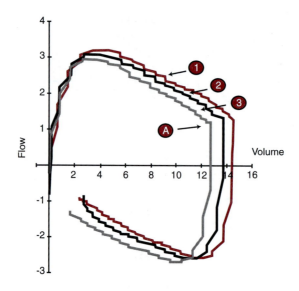

Figure 5-17. Breath-stacking flow-volume loops.

The F-V loops in Figure 5-17 labeled 1, 2, and 3 coincide with the shaded curves on the scalars. Note how each loop has an increase in volume as the mechanical rate is increased and how flow does not reach baseline before the next positive pressure breath is delivered. The P-V loop in Figure 5-18 shows the volume retained in the lung at end-exhalation. Also note how with each successive breath the baseline pressure rises due to the trapped gas in the lung. Observe the large resistance created by breath-stacking.

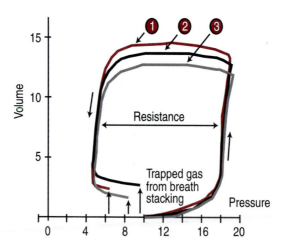

Figure 5-18. Breath-stacking pressure-volume loops.

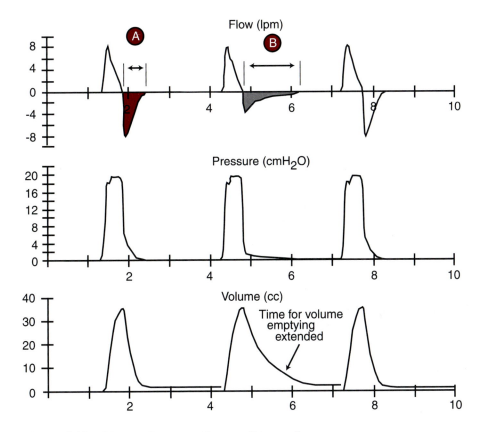

Figure 5-19. Obstruction to expiratory flow scalars.

Compare the shaded expiratory waveforms A and B in Figure 5-19. Waveform A shows a normal expiratory waveform reaching baseline in a short period of time. The expiatory waveform is a mirror image of the inspiratory waveform. In B note how the expiratory waveform is shorter (less flow rate) and the expiratory time is longer. This indicates there is resistance to exhalation. Also note on the volume scalar the shape of the volume scalar as compared to the first volume scalar. The time for volume emptying is longer due to expiratory resistance. Also recognize how the volume baseline is raised compared to the first volume waveform. The second pressure waveform also shows extended time for emptying of the lung. No breath-stacking is seen here in spite of prolonged exhalation due to the long exhalation time set on the ventilator.

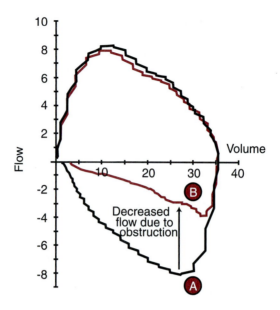

Figure 5-20. Expiratory flow rate obstruction flow-volume loops.

Compare points A and B in the F-V loop shown in Figure 5-20. The inspiratory flow is normal in both A and B. A decrease in expiratory flow rate occurs during grunting and less volume returns at B than at A. The P-V loop in Figure 5-21 shows a widened loop appearance from A to B indicating a greater resistance, due to expiratory grunting. The loop enlargement during exhalation indicates resistance during exhalation.

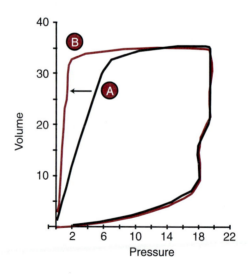

Figure 5-21. Expiratory flow rate obstruction pressure-volume loops.

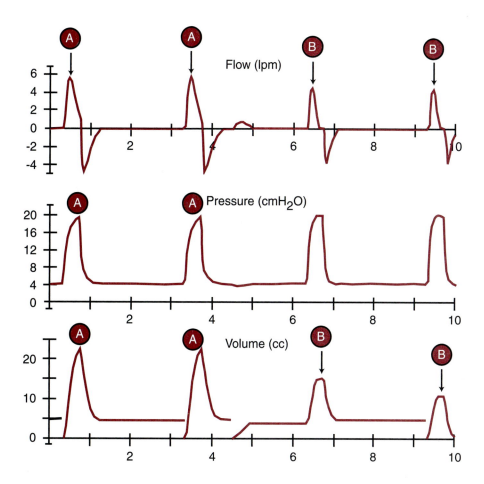

Figure 5-22. Neonatal right mainstem intubation scalars.

The scalars in Figure 5-22 show changes in flow rate and volume as the ET-tube moves from the trachea into the right main stem bronchus. Point A represents normal flow and volume and pressure scalars from proper placement of the ETT. Point B represents the tube having moved into the right main stem bronchus. The volume scalar shows a reduction in volume compared to point A and flow rate is reduced compared to point A. Pressure remains unchanged in this pressure-controlled mode of ventilation.

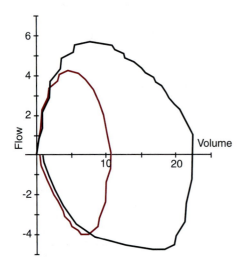

Figure 5-23. Right mainstem bronchus intubation flow-volume loops.

Right mainstem intubation results in a decreased volume and peak flow rate as seen in Figure 5-23. The red loop takes on the typical pattern for a restrictive condition. This is due to the decreased compliance of ventilating one lung.

A change in patient compliance during pressure-targeted ventilation causes change in both pressure and volume. The ventilator adjusts flow rate to maintain a constant pressure as seen in Figure 5-24. A change in patient respiratory system compliance using pressure-targeted ventilation results in a volume change but little change in loop hysteresis.

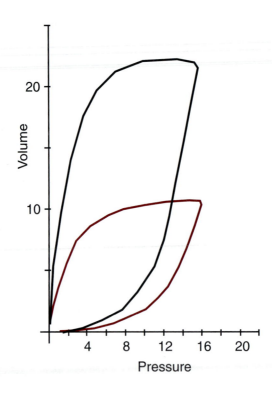

Figure 5-24. Right mainstem bronchus intubation pressure-volume loops.

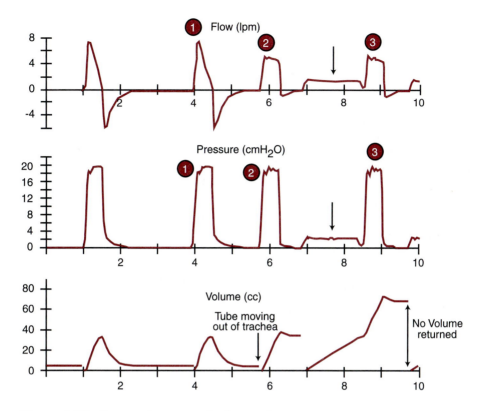

Figure 5-25. Progression to extubation scalars.

Breath 1 on the flow scalar in Figure 5-25 represents a normal condition with the ET-tube positioned through the vocal cords into the trachea. Normal flow rate, pressure, and volume waveforms are seen at this point. As the tube starts to move out of the trachea, note the decrease in returned volumes. With the tube completely out of the trachea no volume is returned. The flow and pressure curves are altered by the reduction in returned volume.

In loop 1 of the F-V loop in Figure 5-26, the ET-tube is in the trachea. Loop 2 represents the ET-tube partially out of the trachea with little volume return seen. Waveform 3 shows increased inspiratory volume with no expiratory volume returning because the tube is completely out of the trachea. The flow and volume changes seen are inherent to the pressure and time constant being maintained throughout breaths even during partial extubation. This is inherent to ventilators in pressure mode settings. Flow is variable as it makes every attempt to hold pressure constant throughout the time constant set on the ventilator in cases of leaks or increased compliance.

Loop 1 of the P-V loops in Figure 5-27 represents the ET-tube in proper position in the trachea. Loop 2 coincides with the ET-tube starting to come out of the trachea. Loop 3 represents the ETT completely out of the trachea with no exhaled volume detected by the monitoring device. The vent-ilator's attempt to maintain a constant baseline pressure in the presence of an overwhelming leak results in the graphics monitor recording an increased inspiratory volume.

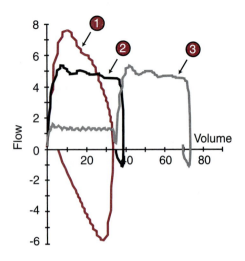

Figure 5-26. Progression to extubation flow-volume loops.

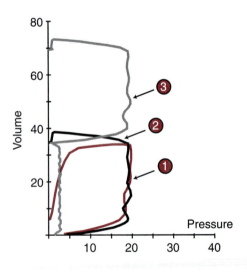

Figure 5-27. Progression to extubation pressure-volume loops.

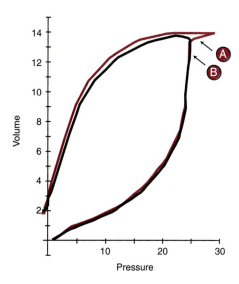

Figure 5-28. Effect of excessive inspiratory pressure on the P-V loop (beaking).

Point A on the P-V curve in Figure 5-28 shows an increase in pressure with no change in volume. This is often referred to as "beaking." At point B the pressure is decreased from 29 cm H2O to 25 cm H2O and the curve has a more rounded appearance at peak inspiration. Although the pressure is reduced there is little change in the delivered volume.

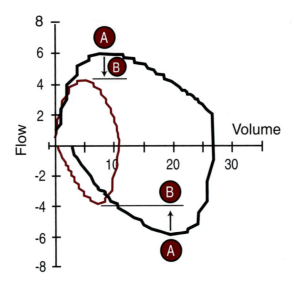

Figure 5-29. Reduced compliance flow-volume loop.

The P-V loop in Figure 5-29 represents a reduction in the lung compliance. Loop A represents a high compliance with a 25 mL of air being delivered. Loop B shows a reduction in compliance where volume delivery is reduced to approximately 10 mL given the same amount of pressure as in loop A. The P-V loop A in Figure 5-30 shows a similar volume as in the F-V loop A in Figure 5-29. The reduction in volume and flow in Figure 5-30 is a consequence of reduced lung compliance.

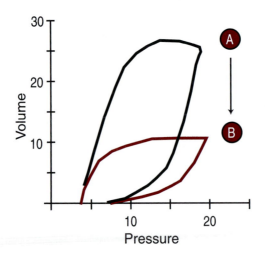

Figure 5-30. Reduced compliance pressure-volume loop.

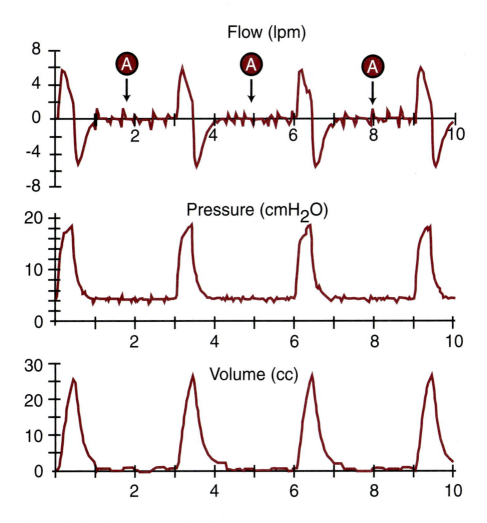

Figure 5-31. Turbulent baseline flow rate scalars.

Water from condensation in the inspiratory limb of the ventilator circuit creates non-uniform waveform appearance in each of the scalars between each positive pressure breath (Figure 5-31). This may also be caused by secretions in the endotracheal tube and airways or water within the inspiratory limb of the patient's circuit.

APPENDIX
CASE STUDIES
NEONATAL CASE STUDY 1

Aaron was born by cesarean section delivery at 26 weeks gestation because of premature rupture of membranes. His mother received prenatal steroids. His Apgar score was
6 and 9 at 1 and 5 minutes respectively. He was resuscitated with positive pressure
ventilation with 100% oxygen. He was intubated with a 2.5 mm ID endotracheal tube,
stabilized, and transported to NICU. His birthweight was 667 grams, birth length 32
cm, head circumference 23.5 cm. He was in the 10th percentile and was small for
gestational age. He was worked up for RDS, sepsis, and patent ductus arteriosus. He
was given gentamicin and ampicillin. Aaron was placed on pressure-limited, time-
cycled, constant flow ventilation with the following settings: PIP 20 cm H_2O, rate 40/
min, inspiratory time 0.3 seconds, F_IO2 0.50, PEEP 5 cm H_2O, IMV mode. Over the
next 3 days Aaron required increases in F_IO2 for desaturation. He appeared restless,
irritable, had pale color, and was tachycardiac. His chest radiograph showed a
reticulogranular appearance in both lungs, signs of pneumothorax, and tube placement was appropriate. Graphic monitoring was begun and the following flow-volume
and pressure-volume loops were obtained.

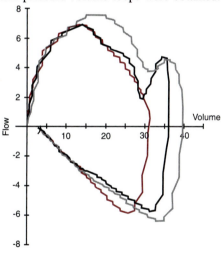
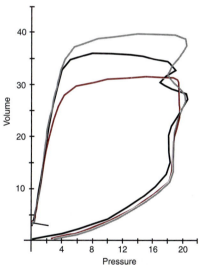

Questions
1.   What do these loop tracings indicate?

After obtaining these loops a ventilator change was made and the following F-V and P-V loops were obtained.

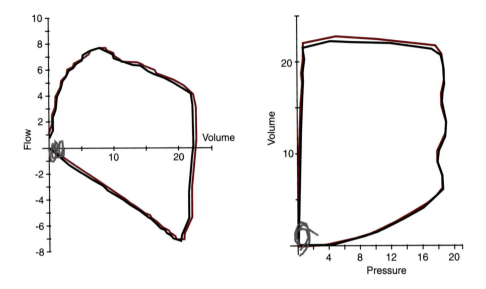

2.   What ventilator setting was changed?

Answers to Neonatal Case Study 1

1.   These loops indicate patient-ventilator asynchrony. Note how on the F-V loop flow increases then decreases twice during the inspiratory phase. The patient initiated another inspiratory effort near the end of the ventilator's inspiratory period. Note the variation in the volume due to the mechanical breath delivered "on top of" the infant's spontaneous breath or the mechanical breath delivered as the infant is exhaling.

2.   Intermittent mandatory ventilation mode was changed to synchronized inter-mittent mandatory ventilation. Note how the breaths are synchronized with the patient's inspiratory effort and that each mechanical breath is nearly the same volume. This mode provided sychronization between patient and ventilator.

NEONATAL CASE STUDY 2

Kristin is a 32 week gestational age infant born by cesarean section. Her mother had a poor biophysical profile and premature rupture of membranes. Her Apgar was 7 and 9 at 1 minute and 5 minutes respectively. She received blow-by oxygen and was suctioned. She was breathing spontaneously and was taken to NICU for observation and septic work up. Six hours later she required intubation and mechanical ventilation. She is currently on pressure-limited, time-cycled, continuous flow ventilation at the following settings: PIP 20 cm H_2O, rate 30/min, PEEP 4 cm H_2O, inspiratory time 0.4 seconds and F_1O2 0.30. After receiving care from her nurse, endotracheal tube suctioning and endotracheal tube retaping from the respiratory care practitioner, she was placed on her stomach with her head turned to the left. After leaving Kristin's bed and closing the isolette the respiratory care practitioner observed the following graphic waveform.

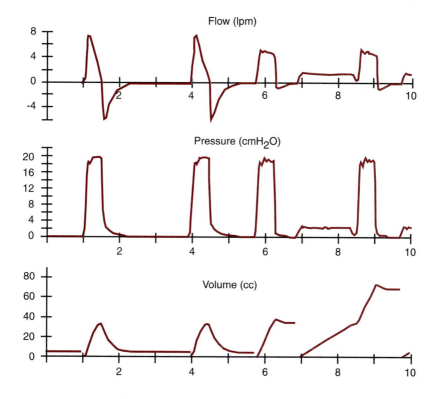

Questions

1.   What do these scalars indicate?

2.   What should be done at this time to correct this situation?

Answers to Neonatal Case Study 2

1.   These scalars indicate that Kristin's endotracheal tube is out of her trachea and above her vocal cords. The first two waveforms on the flow, pressure, and volume scalar represent a normal condition with the endotracheal tube correctly positioned within the trachea. Note the third waveform on the volume scalar. There is less return volume to be registered indicating the tube is above the vocal cords. There is no return volume to be registered by the pneumotach because the inspiratory volume has escaped out through the mouth and nose.

2.   Appropriate treatment at this time would be to look down into Kristin's airway with a laryngoscope to confirm endotracheal tube extubation. Upon confirmation remove the tube, bag-mask ventilate Kristin to stabilize her then reintubate her.

NEONATAL CASE STUDY 3

A 20-year-old gave birth to Rodney, a 27 week, 785 gram baby born by vaginal delivery. The mother had no prenatal care and she had premature rupture of membranes for 3 days prior to delivery. Apgar scores were 5 and 9 at 1 minute and 5 minutes respectively following bag-mask ventilation. Rodney was intubated with a 2.5 mm ID oral endotracheal tube and given one dose of surfactant. Rodney was transferred to NICU and placed on pressure-limited, time-cycled ventilation with the following settings: PIP 20 cm H_2O, rate 40/min, inspiratory time 0.3 seconds, PEEP 5 cm H_2O, F_IO2 1.0. Ten hours after the initial dose of surfactant was given, Rodney exhibited signs of respiratory distress with intercostal and suprasternal retractions, spontaneous respiratory rate increase from 48 to 88/min, pulse increase from 138 to 178/min, and increased periods of desaturation below 90%. Exhaled tidal volume decreased from 5 mL/kg to 2.5 mL/kg. The F_IO2 which was weaned to 0.30 has been increased to 0.70 to maintain saturation above 90%. The following P-V curve (B) was obtained and compared to the P-V curve (A) taken after administration of the initial dose of surfactant.

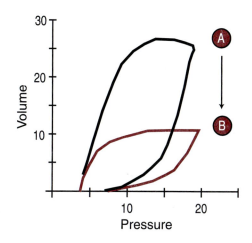

Questions

1.   What has caused the change in the P-V loop between A and B?

2.   Based on P-V loop B what would you recommend at this time?

Answers to Neonatal Case Study 3

1.   The P-V loop change from A to B indicates a decrease in lung compliance. Notice that the pressure remains the same at 20 cm H_2O but the volume decreased from approximately 27 mL to 10 mL. Typically a reduced compliance causes a shift of the P-V loop to the right.

2.   It would be appropriate to administer another dose of surfactant at this time in response to the reduced lung compliance.

ADULT CASE STUDY 1

Joyce is a 40-year-old black female status post motor vehicle accident. After 3 days in the ICU she was being ventilated with volume-targeted SIMV at a V_T of 750 ml, PEEP of 7 cm H_2O, and set frequency of 16 breaths/minute.

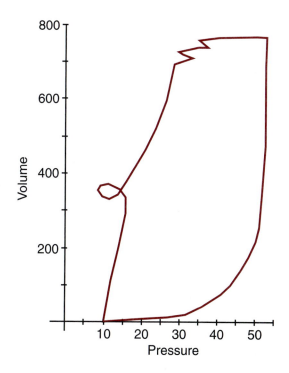

Questions
1.   What is the dynamic compliance for this patient?

2.   What abnormalities are present in the above P-V loop?

In an attempt to better synchronize the ventilator to the patient without sedation, the mode was changed to PSV with a set pressure of 28 cm H_2O. The resulting P-V loop is shown below.

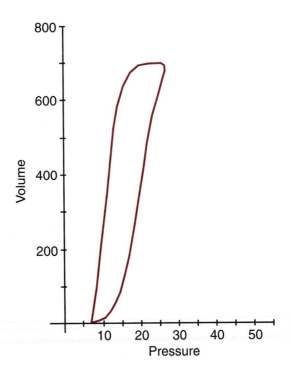

3.   What is the patient's dynamic compliance after the change?

4.   Would this ventilator change be considered an improvement or worsening of the patient's synchrony with the ventilator?

Answers to Adult Case Study 1

1.   The dynamic compliance was approximately 17 ml/cm H_2O.

2.   The P-V loop exhibited increased hysteresis, disruption/dys-synchrony at the beginning of exhalation, and a spontaneous inspiratory effort towards the end of exhalation.

3.   The dynamic compliance was approximately 33 ml/cm H_2O.

4.   For this particular patient, PSV mode improved patient-ventilator synchrony and yielded less loop hysteresis and improved compliance.

ADULT CASE STUDY 2

Albert is a 62-year-old Hispanic male with bilateral pneumonia and a history of asthma. He was intubated four hours ago and was placed on assist control ventilation, peak flow of 70 L/min, descending flow pattern, and PEEP of 6 cm H_2O. The flow-trigger sensitivity was set at 3 L/min. Upon completion of morning rounds the attending physician ordered bronchodilator therapy via small volume nebulizer. After completing the first ventilator check of the shift and performing a brief respiratory assessment, the respiratory therapist started the bronchodilator treatment via the ventilator's built-in nebulizer control and records an initial pair of F-V and P-V loops for pre- and post-bronchodilator comparison. The initial loops are shown below.

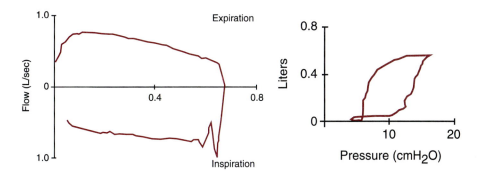

Questions

1. What abnormal findings are present in the F-V loop?

2. What abnormal findings are present in the P-V loop?

Immediately after the conclusion of the treatment the therapist records a pair of post-bronchodilator loops which are shown the next page. Although sufficient time has not passed to properly assess the effect of the bronchodilator, the therapist wanted to see if the previous abnormalities had been at least somewhat improved. Based on comparing the pre-bronchodilator loops to the post-bronchodilator loops, answer the following questions.

3.   Do the loops indicate benefit from the bronchodilator?

4.   Are the other initial abnormalities improved?

5.   What is the source/s of the other abnormalities?

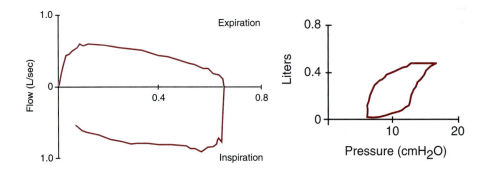

Answers to Adult Case Study 2

1.   The pre-bronchodilator loop has a jagged disruption at the beginning of inspiration that looks similar to dys-synchrony. At the end of inspiration the waveform appears to dead-end and then restart at the horizontal axis for the expiratory phase. Note that the P-V loop is closed (no leak). Some air-trapping may be present.

2.   The inspiratory curve has coarse fluctuations and some overdistension is seen at the end of inspiration. Considerable patient effort (for this compromised patient) is required to trigger the machine breath as evidenced by the prominent leftward bulge at the beginning of inspiration.

3.   Although slight changes can be argued, the loops do not indicate the typical signs of improvement associated with bronchodilator therapy.

4.   The initial inspiratory abnormality is resolved but the end-inspiratory dead-end persists.

5.   The transient problem at the beginning of inspiration was actually a surge of gas flow produced by the ventilator's internal nebulizer compressor. When the ventilator's internal nebulizer function is on, sensitivity is automatically switched to pressure-triggering because flow-triggering cannot be used under that condition. The poor sensitivity problem was due to an inappropriate pressure-trigger setting. The break in the F-V loop tracing at the end of inspiration is not seen in the P-V loop indicating it is not due to a loss of volume. There is likely a problem with the graphic monitor's ability to display this particular condition due to a coordination problem between the ventilator's timing circuit and the F-V data from the transducer.

Index